Assessment and Care Planning in Mental Health Nursing

Assessment and Care Planning in Mental Health Nursing

Nick Wrycraft

Mc Graw Hill Education Open University Press

Open University Press
McGraw-Hill Education
McGraw-Hill House
Shoppenhangers Road
Maidenhead
Berkshire
England
SL6 2QL

email: enquiries@openup.co.uk
world wide web: www.openup.co.uk

and Two Penn Plaza, New York, NY 10121-2289, USA

First published 2015

A catalogue record of this book is available from the British Library

ISBN-13: 978-0-33-526474-2
ISBN-10: 0-33-526474-3
eISBN: 978-0-33-526475-9

Library of Congress Cataloging-in-Publication Data
CIP data applied for

Typeset by Aptara, Inc.
Printed and bound by CPI Group (UK) Ltd, Croydon, CR0 4YY

Praise for this book

"I would highly recommend this book to all mental health nursing students. Whilst the focus is on assessment and care planning, knowledge and skills on a range of essential areas are present in this text. It is an essential handbook for key mental health nursing skills. Case studies are presented with clarity, and Nick Wrycraft is clearly committed to nurses learning from service users, which is essential for values-based practice."

Julia Terry, Senior Lecturer in Mental Health Nursing,
Swansea University, UK

"This text is a good fit for mental health nursing students new to assessment and care planning, providing a practical rather than academic approach to these important aspects of the role."

Dr Janine Archer Lecturer School of Nursing, Midwifery & Social Work,
University of Manchester, UK

Thanks to my wife Alex and children Emily and Hamish for their perseverance and support. Also to Alison Coad for her advice, Gary Morris and Danny Walsh for their comments, and Richard Townrow and Karen Harris for all of their support; also Rachel Crookes for her help in developing the proposal to begin with.

Contents

SECTION 3
Case studies

About the author

Nick Wrycraft is a registered mental health nurse and senior lecturer at Anglia Ruskin University, UK, where he teaches pre-registration nursing. Nick's thesis for his professional doctorate was on clinical supervision in adult nursing primary care settings. His specialist interests include mental health interventions in primary care and mental health promotion. Nick has previously edited *Introduction to mental health nursing* (2009) and *Mental health nursing: case book* (2012), was co-writer with Vanesssa Skinner of *CBT fundamentals: cases and practice* (2014), and co-editor with Alison Coad of *CBT approaches for children and young people* (2015). Currently Nick is working on further collaborative writing projects.

Preface

This book is about assessment and care planning in mental health nursing, and how mental health nurses can gain an understanding of the service user's experience of mental illness. Within the book there are three interlinked aims. We start by considering: what is assessment? Thinking about what assessment really means helps us to understand the role it performs, and enables us to adapt our approach and to carry out better assessments. This is especially useful as often assessment represents the service user's first point of contact with the service and there is the opportunity to encourage engagement and positive perceptions of mental health services as a source of support.

The second aim of the book is to show that assessment ought not to be a stand-alone activity but actively contribute alongside other aspects of the nursing process to the care of service users. In this respect the nursing process is not cyclical but highly fluid, and the stages are mutually interdependent. Assessment informs the planning and implementation of care that follows, and the better the relationship between these two elements of the nursing process the more likely it is that the care plan will be effective and cohesive. The final aim is to encourage reflection upon skills in assessment and care planning, and the cultivation and development of these capabilities as an ongoing and continuous process. We will now briefly consider how these aims have informed the structure of the book.

Section 1 consists of nine brief chapters. In Chapters 1–4 we specifically meet the first aim of the book in the sense of being focused on assessment, although Chapters 2–4 apply to both assessment and care planning. In Chapter 1 we consider a definition of assessment, before considering the approaches that are taken, the techniques and methods, and the values that are important in assessment. Chapter 2 then focuses on communication skills and engagement with the person, and this theme continues, developing into Chapter 3 where we look at empathy and therapeutic rapport. In Chapter 4 we discuss risk, as this forms an important element of all assessment and care planning in mental health nursing.

The second aim of this book is addressed in Chapters 5–8, where we focus upon how the information elicited in assessment is used to devise care plans, before considering working in partnership, interventions and relapse prevention in terms of being inextricably linked to assessment and forming part of a cohesive and interlinked process. Finally, in Chapter 9 we meet the third aim of the book, and focus upon reflection and learning from experience in carrying out assessment and care planning, as well as looking at how we might further develop.

In Section 2 we discuss some specific features of mental health problems that are commonly evident. The approach that has been taken purposely does not use standardized diagnostic terms. The reason for this is to avoid stereotyping, and the use of cliché-ridden understandings of mental health problems that often miss the individual nuances of personal experience. The section is organized into four chapters that conform to the stages of the cognitive behavioural model which is the most commonly used evidence-based model within the mental health field. These are: behaviours, feelings, thoughts and physical features. The mental health issues covered in these chapters are broken down under the headings of: definition/context, engagement, assessment, care planning, intervention, relapse management and then further reading.

Finally, Section 3 provides practical examples of how prioritized needs that emerge from assessment are translated into care planned goals and suggested interventions in four detailed case studies and comprehensive care plans.

Introduction

Assessment and care planning are essential aspects of mental health nursing. Yet in order to carry these out effectively a range of skills are required. These include an understanding of the concepts of assessment and care planning, and how they contribute to nursing care, an appreciation of the principles of professional practice and ethical awareness, as well as communication and interpersonal skills. All of these aspects interweave seamlessly together in assisting the mental health nurse in carrying out effective assessments and planning person-centred care.

The intention of this book is to encourage you to consider what assessment and care planning are, and their purpose and role in mental health nursing. Yet also to reflect upon the wide range of skills that are involved, and your own personal approach in carrying out these activities in a manner that genuinely engages with the service user, and accurately captures the nature of their needs.

First it is necessary to decide what we expect of assessment. In contemplating this issue it helps to reflect on how well can we ever know anyone. Consider your answer for a few seconds. It is tempting to think that especially concerning those to whom we are closest, such as family, relatives and friends, and with whom we spend much of our time, we know them to the extent that in most circumstances we can predict their responses. While this might be true for the majority of the time, it is also the case that there always remains the potential for them to surprise us, and to defy our expectations. In fact there is only so much that we can know about anyone. While this may seem to be a pessimistic conclusion, what attracts many of us to working with people is the constant capacity for surprise. We are aware of how little we know about people, and are curious to know more. Our expectations of assessment therefore need to be tempered with an awareness of the limitations of what we can claim to know. Furthermore, it is also necessary to recognize and put aside our preconceptions and assumptions. Assessment is about hearing the person's individual story, and appreciating how they experience the issues in their lives and make sense of their situation.

Our expectation and understanding of assessment has implications for how we view the role that it performs in mental health nursing practice. The greatest emphasis on assessment tends to be during the service user's first meeting with the mental health nurse, or, for example, during the first few days of their inpatient admission. Although mental health nursing assessments occur in a variety of situations, often they are in a hospital ward, or an environment that is busy and unfamiliar to the person. Furthermore, they are also frequently time limited, and there may be some specific mandatory questions that need to be answered. All of this also occurs when the person is acutely distressed, or in crisis. These factors compromise the mental health nurse's capacity to engage effectively with the person, form a therapeutic rapport, and really gain an understanding of their situation. Instead, and if assessments are to be really effective, multiple meetings may need to occur over time, to gain a broad and truly representative picture of the person and their needs. Therefore assessment is a specific activity carried out over a prolonged period, as opposed to a snapshot taken early on during a person's initial contact with the service.

Care planning is the other focal point of this book, and has equal emphasis in the other stages of the nursing process. In practice, students find this stage hard to identify, as they do not see it happening as a specific event, or at a particular place and time. While activity related to assessment is frequently flagged up and readily apparent, in contrast care planning is more discreet and occurs in many different places and settings. These include multidisciplinary meetings, and discussions between teams and individuals, the writing-up of assessments and completing documentation, as well as discussions with service users, their carers, significant others and family members.

Furthermore, if care planning is to produce effective and meaningful goals and outcomes then this requires agreement between the mental health nurse and the service user. Yet frequently the service user has come into contact with mental health services precisely because they do not agree with the professionals' perceptions of their problems. This means that often discussion of the care plan is characterized by disagreement. These differences may therefore be seen as representing disruptions to the smooth flow of the care planning stage of the nursing process and the therapeutic relationship, and to undermine mental health nursing theory.

Instead, these developments ought to be seen as an inextricable part of planning care. In this book care planning is discussed in terms of several separate stages and points within the overall care process. This reflects the gradual process of discussion, negotiation and collaboration between the mental health nurse and the service user as it is found in practice. Differences between the nurse and the service user can be seen as characterizing what happens in the planning of care, and rather than representing an obstacle to care it is how these are skilfully addressed by the mental health nurse that is central to the discussion.

Perhaps the most important factor that holds everything else together is that in assessment and the planning of care a range of interpersonal and communication skills are used based upon positive values. These contribute to the development of a trusting therapeutic rapport that places the person at their ease and helps them feel accepted and supported, and also has the potential to perform a therapeutic role. Although mental health nursing students often describe themselves as 'people-orientated' (which is why they choose to enter the profession) it is then blithely assumed that these skills will naturally develop further into professional values. Instead, and to transform an inclination towards working with people into a professional principle that finds expression in practice, consciously focused learning and reflection is required in order to develop self-awareness.

Yet examining our own preconceptions is challenging and difficult to do, while acknowledging our own shortcomings, limitations and learning needs can make people feel vulnerable, and even lead to their resorting to defence mechanisms. Central to achieving this transformation is for student mental health nurses to actively seek to develop trusting and open relationships with lecturers, mentors in clinical practice and their peers, be receptive to feedback and have a commitment to learning.

Finally, assessment and care planning occur in a political context and in recent years mental health services have experienced a straitening of resources. As a result there is less service provision overall, and people are often already in crisis before coming into contact with mental health services. Furthermore, there is a lack of specialist provision for some groups such as children and younger people with mental health issues, while those with complex mental health issues and people with dual diagnosis often fall outside the strict remits of those specialist services that do exist. Consequently, many people with complex and severe mental health issues are within mainstream mental health services, where it is of little surprise that some – for example, those with personality disorders – become unpopular with overstretched staff that lack the specialist skills required to work effectively with their issues. These challenging factors are often viewed negatively. However, a realistic consequence for mental health nurses is that within these difficult settings effective assessment skills are needed more than ever and are in constant use. These skills include developing and continuously updating a sound knowledge base and understanding of mental health practice. Equally important is to develop effective communication and interpersonal skills based on positive values. Through adopting an approach that combines these elements it is possible to carry out assessment and care planning that focuses upon the person and their needs and concerns, while also demonstrating care, compassion and humanity.

Initiating relationships with service users and conducting assessments

1   Assessment in mental health

Introduction

In this chapter we will consider what assessment is in the context of the nursing process, and the stages of which it is composed, before discussing why we carry out assessments. We then focus on approaches to assessment, including interviews, observations and assessment tools. The chapter then moves on to discuss the techniques used in assessment, including sight and smell, verbal and non-verbal assessment, instinct, communication skills and open and closed questions. Finally we will consider the way the assessments we make will be informed by our personal values.

By the end of this chapter the reader will have:

- considered a definition of assessment
- understood approaches to assessment
- gained an insight into techniques of assessment
- appreciated the contribution of values in assessment.

A definition and understanding of assessment

Assessment in mental health nursing is often seen as part of a process composed of assessment, planning, implementation and evaluation (APIE). Sometimes an additional stage of diagnosis is identified between the assessment and planning stages. Yet this could be seen as making mental health nursing biomedical, and undermining the more psychosocial aspect of mental health assessments.

While the nursing process provides a useful framework for the delivery of care and setting goals for progress, it can also lead to the unrealistic perception of nursing as only occurring within a process of neat and equal stages. In practice the stages of the nursing process often occur simultaneously or overlap, and furthermore we also ought to be assessing throughout the whole process. Therefore it is more accurate to see the individual stages of the nursing process as complementary and mutually informative, as opposed to forming a sequential cycle. Therefore in this book we consider assessment as inextricably linked to other parts of the nursing process to create cohesive, comprehensive and personalized care for the service user.

Q: Why do we assess? Write down a list of the reasons why we carry out assessments and then compare what you have written with the answers below.

A: *To understand the nature, extent and severity to which the person is affected by their mental health problems.*
  To identify what services or therapeutic interventions might best fit the person's needs.
  To carry out baseline measurements against which to make later comparisons to be able to monitor progress and to recognize patterns, changes and improvements in the person's mental health.
  To gain information for the completion of documentation and paperwork in accordance with legal and organizational requirements.
  To practise in accordance with professional standards of healthcare, practitioners need to carry out assessments before working with service users.
  Because having the opportunity to speak about and explain the problem in their own words is often empowering and therapeutic for the person.

All of the above are reasons why we might carry out an assessment.

In assessment, the mental health nurse attempts to form an understanding of the person's situation and the circumstances that contribute to their health status. **Assessment** is the purposeful gathering of relevant information to form a comprehensive understanding of the person's mental, physical and sociological health.

Yet too much emphasis upon any aspect of the biological, psychological and sociological perspectives of health provides only a partial understanding of the issue, as people do not experience problems in just one area of their life. Instead it is often the case, for example, that a physical health issue will impact upon the person's psychological and sociological well-being. For each of us this combination of factors will be different.

Therefore assessment has two distinct stages. These are:

- the **collection of data** in the form of biological, psychological and sociological information about the person
- the **interpretation of this data** to establish a profile of the person and their mental health.

In this sense assessment is like a prism, through which the individual colours within white light can be seen. When carrying out an assessment we can understand more about the different bio-psychosocial factors at work in the person's life and how these combine, interact and influence their mental health and well-being.

In carrying out assessment, each new conversation is a different event, and it is necessary to avoid imposing our expectations and values on the person and their situation. Instead assessment is the opportunity to understand the service user's

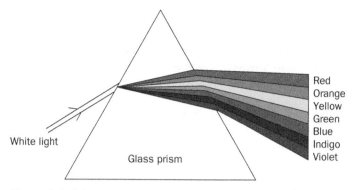

Figure 1.1 Prism

sense of their experience and the events in their life from their perspective, and in terms of their priorities as the expert in their health. In this respect in assessment our focus must be intently on the service user and committed to learning from them. Furthermore, assessment is not just about looking for the detrimental effects of mental ill-health but also for the person's capabilities, positive coping resources, strengths and skills. The areas that assessment covers might include:

- identifying the nature and extent of the problem(s) and impact upon the person
- psychological strengths, abilities and coping resources
- what is important to the person
- the person's values and beliefs
- their quality of life
- their cultural and ethnic values
- their family and social network
- their background and upbringing
- their choice of lifestyle
- their education and financial situation
- their current mood
- their motivation
- their mental state
- risk
- physical health, well-being and resilience
- the capacity to live independently
- past experiences of healthcare.

When conducting an assessment it is important that we know exactly why we are collecting the information in order to avoid:

- being unnecessarily intrusive
- asking irrelevant questions
- focusing on the wrong areas of investigation.

We should always reflect on the following questions:

- What is the intended purpose of the information being collected?
- Does the information usefully add to what is already known?
- Is this an appropriate or relevant area of investigation?

Within the two stages of assessment identified above, data is first collected in its entirety before any interpretations are made. Following this approach avoids drawing premature and possibly mistaken conclusions. Through observing these stages, mental health nursing assessments will be as accurate as possible and practice will be guided by evidence, as we are forming conclusions based on all of the available information.

Considering these factors will allow us to plan assessments that are focused and generate information that is useful in helping to plan the person's care. Next we will look at the approaches that are used in carrying out assessment.

Approaches to assessment

Approaches to assessment fall into three general categories. These are the comprehensive interview, observations and focused assessment tools.

- The comprehensive **interview** covers all aspects of the person's bio-psychosocial functioning and is often carried out, for example, when a person is admitted to an inpatient ward. A meeting will be held with the person and their background and health profile will be discussed in detail. A comprehensive physical health assessment will also be carried out with a doctor.
- **Observations** of a person's actions, manner, behaviour and speech might be used, for example, on an inpatient unit to assess the person's mood on a regular basis as part of an ongoing assessment. However, it is also possible for these to be used in the community, where the mental health nurse will routinely observe and assess the person's mental state to identify improvement or deterioration. The assessment will also consider other aspects of self-care such as:
  - hygiene
  - nutrition and hydration
  - lifestyle and recent changes to the person's pattern of living
  - social and economic factors
  - any use of substances or alcohol and the effects of these.
- **Assessment tools** can be used that focus on a particular phenomenon or aspect of functioning. Assessment tools commonly consist of a number of specific, fixed-answer questions and the responses are then scored to reveal a total indicating the person's level of functioning at that point in time. Often the initial score is used as a baseline and the use of the tool is later repeated to ascertain improvement or deterioration. There are a wide variety of assessment tools which are used for many aspects of a person's bio-psychosocial functioning.

Elsewhere in this book we discuss observation and assessment tools in more depth. For the moment we will focus on interviews, as these are often the first point of contact with the person and are an intensive method of data collection, involving a high level of interpersonal skills and self-awareness. We will look at the overall approaches that are taken, before focusing in more detail on the types of questions and techniques that are used.

Interviews can be formal or informal. **Formal interviews** are structured, often flow in a logical sequence and have a specific, time-limited duration. The interviewer and interviewee have defined roles with clear boundaries and specific questions are asked. In some cases the meeting will commence with a discussion of the agenda of issues to be covered and at the end there will be a summary and further actions and outcomes identified together with who is responsible for carrying these out.

In contrast **informal interviews** are often free-flowing and fluid discussions. There will still be a beginning, middle and end to the discussion with some outcomes or actions emerging, but to an observer an informal interview might even appear to resemble a casual conversation. However, this does not appreciate the high level of skill that the interviewer uses to elicit the information that is required while maintaining an informal approach.

Many interviews will combine elements of both the formal and informal interview. While on practice placements it is helpful when attending or participating in assessments to reflect on the type of interview which has been chosen, the reasons why and whether the methods chosen were successful (see Chapter 9 for a wider discussion on reflection).

Q: Below, three reasons have been provided for choosing formal and informal interviews. Of these, one is incorrect. Consider each reason and identify the one that is incorrect. A formal interview might be chosen:

1 Because the person is acutely anxious and has not previously been in contact with mental health services. A formal interview allows the person to understand what will happen next and helps to empower them.
2 Because there is a lot of paperwork and questions to cover and this will help the assessor.
3 Because the person has difficulty focusing their attention. A formal assessment will help the person to focus.

An informal interview might be chosen:

1 Because the person is suspicious and resentful of mental health services. An informal approach might reduce the level of formality within the assessment and be more likely to ensure that the person being assessed engages with the assessment.
2 Because the person is acutely emotionally distressed. An informal assessment and a focus on developing therapeutic rapport is preferable to conducting a formal interview.
3 Because the assessor prefers this type of assessment and has always done it this way.

A: In the case of the formal interview the incorrect reason is 2. The choice of assessment method ought not to be determined by the needs of the service. In the case of the informal interview the incorrect answer is 3. One reason why this answer is incorrect is the same as for the formal interview. However the assessor's being habituated to one type of assessment and being reluctant to change reflects a ritualistic attitude to practice and a reluctance to learn new skills and innovative practice. All of the other four reasons are correct because they have been chosen based on the needs of the service user and to help them better engage in the process.

Regardless of whether a formal or informal approach has been taken, there are common elements in an effective interview.

Q: What might happen in a good interview?

A: There have been introductions and explanations of their reason for the interview and the possible outcome(s) have been explained.
The person being assessed has been listened to and given time to explain their story.
The person feels that their story has been heard and understood.
The interviewer has displayed an awareness of the feelings, emotions and values which the person has towards what is being discussed.
At the end of the assessment there is a summary of the discussion.
In both formal and informal interviews, there will be some actions or outcomes and both parties will understand what happens next.

Q: Reflect on situations in practice where you have witnessed a good interview. What made it so good? Are there any techniques that you might be able to add to your own approach?

Techniques of assessment

Q: What different techniques might we use to collect information in assessment?

A: The techniques commonly used to collect information include:
- assessment tools in relation to specific aspects of the person's functioning
- observation of the person's actions, mood, manner, behaviour and orientation to the environment that might occur either over time or during one meeting
- questions based on the requirements of an assessment form and gaps in our understanding of the person's situation
- discussion with the person and their significant others
- the overall impressions of the assessor.

Although in many clinical settings familiar formats are often used, there is no such thing as a standard assessment as all people are different and unique and the process of assessment ought to be regarded as new each time, so that we are able to engage with and effectively assess the person. The range of techniques that we use to collect and receive information ought to make optimal use of our senses and reflect the full range of skills evident in everyday communication. These include:

- **Visual senses** and information derived from observing the person. This applies to behaviour, mood and manner but also to clothing and style of dress. If the assessment is in the person's home the assessor will form an impression of the person from their environment and their possessions. For example, if the person has numerous family photographs on prominent display this may indicate a close attachment to and prioritization of their relatives.

- **Olfactory senses** in the form of smell will tell us whether the person is taking care of their personal hygiene but also in some cases whether the person has a physical health problem.
- **Non-verbal interaction** in the person's gestures, behaviour and body language and whether they are expressive or lacking in animation. In some cases it may be necessary to consider cultural influences and these can be varied and subtle.
- **Verbal interaction** and the content and manner of the person's speech.
- **Instinct** and the feeling that the assessor has about the person's circumstances. Numerous terms are applied to this factor including: hunch, instinct, gut feeling and intuition. In all cases it is worth while considering what evidence supports this feeling and impression and how it might be described to a sceptical colleague to clarify the accuracy of and the reasons supporting the assessor's perceptions.

All of these different aspects contributed to the assessments carried out in the case studies in Section 3, and combine to create the impression the mental health nurse forms of the person and their mental health problem. Often assessment will involve the use of multiple techniques that are then cross-referenced to represent a profile of the person

In interviews the most frequently used technique will be questions, either closed or open.

Closed questions have fixed answers, for example *yes* and *no* or a very limited range of responses. Closed questions often pertain to *facts* about the person.

Q: Can you think of some closed questions?

A: *Closed questions tend to be very specific and factual. Examples include:*
- *Did you have a wash when you got up this morning?*
- *Did you put on clean clothes today?*
- *Where do you live?*
- *How old are you?*
- *What is your name?*

Closed questions are quick to answer and provide clear information. They are useful:

- where the same information is sought from many people, for example in a standardized interview
- at the beginning of an interview, as a means of gathering background information about the person
- in certain circumstances where the person is willing to participate but is particularly cautious about providing large amounts of personal detail.

However, closed questions can seem to be quite direct and formal, and this approach can seem insensitive and impersonal and limit the formation of an effective rapport.

In contrast, **open questions** have a wider range of responses and do not have set answers. In many cases open questions enquire about personal experience, opinions or preferences.

Q: Can you think of any open questions?

A: Open questions often do not have 'right' or 'wrong' answers. Examples of open questions are:
- How is your mood today?
- Can you describe your journey here today?
- How do you feel about being here today?
- When you feel down, how do you cheer yourself up?
- What things do you/did you enjoy doing?

Open questions are useful for:

- gaining an insight into the person's viewpoint

- encouraging the person to think about their life and perhaps recall events that they might have thought they had forgotten
- developing a good therapeutic rapport.

However, there is the potential for open questions to delve too deeply into personal feelings and emotions and so they require sensitive use. It is worth remembering the purpose of the assessment is to gain information on the person's mental health and not for the exercise of the interviewer's personal curiosity.

Often an interview will consist of both closed and open questions. For example, we might begin with a series of closed questions. In this way the person being assessed can become acquainted with telling the interviewer about themselves. Because the information being sought is often quite factual, such as the person's preferred name, their date of birth, where they went to school and where they have lived, this is not too intrusive. As the interview progresses, more open questions might be asked in order to learn more about the person's feelings, attitudes and motivations, increasing the depth of the interview.

Values in assessment

In this chapter we have looked at what assessment is and the approaches and techniques that are used. The chapters that follow will go on to consider communication and interpersonal skills, and engagement with the person in assessment. However, what unifies and informs all of these actions, and assessment as a whole, is **values-based practice**.

In simple terms values are beliefs. Every assessment is a new and unique set of interactions and the effectiveness of each assessment relies on the use of a range of skills. The following values should inform all assessments.

Every person's story is unique and individual and has worth and meaning: the person's background is not just a collection of facts but the sum of their personal experiences which have value and meaning (Barker, 2004). The person will have their own understanding of their life events which might be different to what we expect or predict, and so we should avoid making assumptions. The person may also have values that differ from, or even contradict, ours, and so it is important to avoid judging but instead to try and understand the person's point of view if we are to effectively engage with them.

Commit time to the assessment: it is important to prioritize the assessment, to make sure that the time that is promised is spent on the assessment and that we give our undivided attention (Barker, 2004).

The assessment is for the person being assessed: the assessment needs to reflect the preference(s), viewpoint(s) and priorities of the person being assessed and clearly be *for them*. Wherever possible the service user's own words need to be used in describing their experience(s) and wishes.

The assessment needs to be collaborative: the assessment should be shared between the assessor and the person and be a collaborative partnership with shared responsibilities. This may involve patience and giving the person time to make choices and decisions, but is important to ensure that they take ownership of their care.

Be honest at all times: it is necessary for mental health nurses to always tell the truth. At times this might be difficult, however it is important to impart information in a manner that, while clear, is still tactful and discreet.

If we promise something, make sure that we deliver it: it is important that if we say we will carry out an action, we follow it up and let the person know the outcome. Lightly given promises can fundamentally undermine a relationship but being committed to following up actions will mean that we are regarded as reliable and trustworthy and have the person's interests at heart.

Focus on the person's positive coping resources: often assessments can focus on the negative aspects of the person's situation, or the nature of the problem. Identifying the person's achievements, skills and capabilities, no matter how small, offers positive support and avoids a relentlessly negative perspective.

While different values will be more or less apparent depending upon the nature of the assessment and the person's issues, nevertheless they are all relevant and ought always to be considered when carrying out assessments in mental health nursing.

Conclusion

In this chapter we have considered what assessment in mental health nursing is, why we carry out assessment, and the approaches and techniques that we might use. We have also considered the kind of values that underpin what we are doing when we carry out an assessment. While assessments in mental health nursing happen in many different clinical environments, from inpatient areas to the community, there are common values that apply, wherever they occur.

The nature of mental health means that in assessment there is significant emphasis on communicating and engaging with the person in order to elicit the nature of the issue, and even whether the service user perceives there to be a problem. In the following chapters we will look at the use of communication and interpersonal skills to promote engagement with the person.

Reference

Barker, P. (2004) *Assessment in psychiatric and mental health nursing*, 2nd edn. Cheltenham: Nelson Thornes.

Further reading

Aggleton P. and Chalmers, H. (2000) *Nursing models and nursing practice*. 2nd edn. Basingstoke: Macmillan.

Hughes, C., Herron, S. and Younge, J. (2014) *CBT for mild to moderate depression: a guide to low intensity intervention*. Maidenhead: Open University Press.

Gamble, C. and Brennan, G. (2006) Assessments: A rationale for choosing and using, in C. Gamble and G. Brennan (eds) *Working with serious mental illness: a manual for clinical practice*, 2nd edn, pp. 111–30. Philadelphia, PA: Butterworth-Heinemann/Elsevier.

nidirect government services (2014) Mental health assessments, www.nidirect.gov.uk/mental-health-assessments, accessed 9 December 2014.

Royal College of Nursing (2004) Nursing assessment and older people: A Royal College of Nursing toolkit, www.rcn.org.uk/_data/assets/pdf_file/0010/78616/002310.pdf, accessed 9 December 2014.

Walker, S., Carpenter, D. and Middlewick, Y. (2013) *Assessment and decision-making in mental health nursing*, London: Learning Matters.

Ward, M. (1995) *Nursing the psychiatric emergency*. Oxford: Butterworth- Heinemann.

2 Communication and interpersonal skills in assessment

Introduction

In order to make the best possible use of assessment it is necessary to develop effective communication and interpersonal skills to engage with the person. In this chapter and Chapter 3 we will look at these skills, how we use them and how we can develop them further. In achieving this, it is important that we are able to adapt and learn from different situations and challenges that come up in our work. Paying careful attention to how we communicate, the techniques that we use and how we respond to service users will improve our self-awareness, skills and effectiveness in a variety of circumstances.

By the end of this chapter the reader will:

- understand definitions of communication and interpersonal skills
- be able to identify how to begin communicating with people they are assessing
- have considered how to use communication and interpersonal skills in assessment.

Communication and interpersonal skills

Communication can be verbal or non-verbal in form, and is understood as having two quite different functions.

First, communication has the function of sending a message to a recipient and imparting information. To be effective it is necessary for the recipient to understand the message that is being conveyed and to communicate back to the message sender. Communication is therefore a two-way process and an exchange of communication so there are a variety of factors that can determine whether the intended message is received correctly, or misconstrued. Second, and of perhaps greater importance, communication fulfils our inherent need to engage socially with other people, and has a wide range of functions. These include sharing our emotions, impressions, thoughts and ideas. In doing this there can also be a sense of social cohesion, and of belonging, identity, worth and value. Ideas and innovations are shared and developed, while differences are explored, negotiated and mediated. Through communication a sense of culture and shared purpose is derived and maintained, and social rules are negotiated.

Assessment in mental health nursing utilizes both of the above understandings of communication, in not only imparting and receiving information but also demonstrating openness and a willingness to discuss and share information. Effectively communicating with the person and understanding how they *feel* about what they are saying is as important as *what* they are saying. This requires a complex and varied range of verbal and non-verbal skills, as well as positive attitudes and values, which we discussed at the end of the previous chapter.

Q: What is an interpersonally skilled person?

A: **Interpersonal skills** are elusive to define but involve the ability to communicate effectively with other people. An interpersonally skilled person is able to vary their style of communication to meet the needs of the person, or audience, with whom they are interacting. For example, at a multidisciplinary meeting, a mental health nurse may speak to a group of other healthcare professionals, using very specific technical terms and engaging in a vigorous debate, where the mutual parties may robustly disagree with other people's opinions, and articulately present their own views in a forthright and assertive manner. Alternatively, when communicating with a service user who finds it hard to understand complex language, the mental health nurse may avoid technical language and speak in layman's terms, progressing the discussion at a patient, graduated pace that matches the person's capacity to absorb information. There may also be regular pauses to check that the information has been understood, and opportunities for the person to ask questions.

Interpersonal skills require sensitivity to the needs and preferences of others, both verbally and in non-verbal interaction. These needs may not be expressed overtly, as often people feel self-conscious or embarrassed about what they may regard as limitations in their ability to communicate. The mental health nurse needs to be perceptive and observant in picking up clues that will better help them to communicate and engage.

Yet communication is also an active process which requires participation and involvement of the parties involved. In mental health nursing, conversations will often focus on seeking the person's consent to treatment or interventions where they may be reluctant. In this situation, discussing, explaining and negotiating is an essential part of this process, and a purpose in itself, as opposed to the endpoint of securing the person's agreement. In these discussions it is important to demonstrate respect for the person and their viewpoint and to take account of their perspective. For example, in the case of a person who is reluctant to take medication for their mental health, they may believe the medication produces unpleasant side effects and the conversation may consider the nature and severity of the side effects, how long they have been experienced and whether these experiences are in fact due to the medication. It is important that the mental health nurse demonstrates concern for the person and an interest in their situation, and values their views, as opposed to simply ensuring that the person agrees with the need for them to take their medication. Therefore, interpersonal skills overlap with verbal and non-verbal communication, and are held together and supported by being informed by positive values.

Communication covers a wide range of differing functions, which is perhaps why it is so hard to define what makes an interpersonally skilled person. Perhaps we know an interpersonally skilled person when we meet one, and are even more aware when we meet with a person who lacks interpersonal skills.

Q: What range of activities does communication include? Write a list of the different forms of communication you use when you meet with someone, then see how many you identified in the list below.

A: *Communication can take the form of:*
- *attitude: whether we appear interested and receptive to communicating with the person*
- *verbal comments in the form of the words we use*
- *verbal gestures in the sounds we make*
- *non-verbal gestures: deliberate body movements, such as nodding of the head or hand gestures*
- *facial gestures and expressions*
- *eye contact*
- *body posture*
- *proximity to the person*
- *all of the above in various combinations.*

Q: Which of the above aspects do you find difficult or challenging? Make a mental note of an area where you might improve your communication skills and think about ways in which you might carry out practical tasks to overcome this limitation.

Communication is also apparent in terms of the clothing that we wear and the decisions we make about our appearance – for example, hairstyle and colour, tattoos or piercings. As healthcare professionals, it is helpful to consciously reduce the influence that our self-expression might exert on the person being assessed, and to dress inconspicuously – for example by ensuring that tattoos are covered by clothing and piercings are removed while on duty.

Communication also includes the '4WFINDS' questions of what, when, where and with whom (Skinner and Wrycraft, 2014). Often the 4WFINDS are used to help the person that is being assessed to identify factors that are active in situations which cause them problems (see avoidance in behaviours, Chapter 11 pp. 103–6). However, the multi-faceted nature of this framework also makes it a useful method for examining how we might approach an assessment.

- **What?** Do we know what the problem is? There may be a referral, or some description of why the person is being assessed. Sometimes, during the assessment, the problem may emerge as being very different from that described in the referral. It may even be that other problems, outside the referral, are focused on. However, it is necessary to be aware of why the assessment is being carried out.
- **When?** Has the person received suitable advance notice and been advised of any information or paperwork that they may need to bring with them to the assessment – for example, details of any medication they may be prescribed? When using standard letters, it is helpful to closely check the information for accuracy and relevance to the person. Also, is the assessment at a convenient time in relation to the person's normal daily pattern – for example, if the person struggles to attend early appointments can the assessment be scheduled for later in the day?

- **Where?** Is there a suitable room available which: 1) is private and where the assessor and person being assessed can speak confidentially without distraction by noise? 2) is in good decorative repair and suitably furnished? 3) has suitable lighting and ventilation?
- **With whom?** Has the person being assessed been permitted the opportunity to bring someone with them for support if they wish? Will there be many professionals present, and if so has the person been advised that they will be there? Are these professionals known to the person?

Communication in assessment

Q: What preparations can we make before we meet the person that might help us communicate better in an assessment?

A:
- *Know about any specific requirements that may need to be taken into account regarding communication and have made suitable adjustments. For example, does the person speak English? If not, a translator may be needed. Alternatively, if the person has a known hearing deficit we may need to speak clearly with our face visible to the person to supplement our audible communication.*
- *In most assessments the service user will feel some degree of anxiety or nervousness. While this will be more the case for some people than others, nevertheless being prepared for the fact that the person may feel this way will better help the mental health nurse to support the person, should these feelings influence how the person is in the assessment.*
- *Have thoroughly read the person's previous case notes or, if these are unavailable, the referral, and, as in the 'what' of the 4WFINDS questions above, be aware of **what the purpose of the assessment is**. This avoids the person needing to offer lengthy explanations of facts that have previously been identified and instead allows the assessment to focus on their current experience.*

Sometimes before an assessment it is the assessor who feels apprehensive, which can lead to their body language becoming stilted and tense. Or they may come across as overassertive, which can negatively influence the assessment.

Q: What steps can you take to ease your apprehension?

A: *It helps to:*
- *recognize any feelings of tension or anxiety*
- *focus on relaxing thoughts or ideas*
- *consider what will be discussed in the assessment and the strategies that will be used to engage with the person.*

There is no script or recommended formulation of words to use in communicating with the service user during an assessment. Each assessment is a new experience and an authentic, genuine and live encounter during which thought and active participation is required – which is an advantage of the interview approach.

From the outset it is helpful to recognize our impressions of the person, yet also to be wary of jumping to conclusions. As a guide, at the beginning of an assessment, it is necessary to:

- introduce yourself
- state your role
- explain the purpose of the assessment
- explain the intended duration
- explain the possible outcomes
- ask whether the person has any questions.

The language used needs to be simple and straightforward, and avoid jargon. We might then ask: 'Are you okay speaking to me?' This empowers the person and demonstrates a concern for their wishes.

Consider this scenario. **Example 1:** a person has been referred to mental health services due to apparent memory problems. At the beginning of the assessment the mental health nurse asks whether the person would like to take off their coat. Instead the person reaches down to a nearby coffee table where there is an open box of tissues, takes a tissue and offers it to the mental health nurse.

Q: What might the mental health nurse think and how might this influence their communication with the person?

A: *The person appearing to not understand the question does not necessarily prove that they are experiencing a memory problem. There may be other explanations for the person's response, for example:*

- *hearing problems*
- *difficulty with understanding other people's patterns of speech or accents*
- *a physical problem, such as delirium or a urinary tract infection (UTI) that might lead the person to experience confusion or difficulty understanding communication.*

If a comprehensive assessment is being carried out, a physical assessment will also be made and it will be ascertained whether the person has a hearing deficit. Tests would then be carried out to identify any physical causes for the person experiencing memory problems.

Where we doubt the person's capacity, or feel that they are experiencing mental ill-health to the point of their being at risk to themselves or others, we may also need to seek advice and to consider the following legislation:

- the Mental Capacity Act (2005)
- the Mental Health Act (1983 reviewed 2007).

In the assessment we will seek further information as to how the person receives and interprets information and forms their response. Discussion during the assessment should reveal any difficulties they may be experiencing, as will their responses to certain key questions. For example:

- Does the person appear to be consistently muddled or confused? If they appear confused at other times than when answering questions or in conversation, this might confirm that this is not due, for example, to a hearing deficit.
- Does the person retain eye contact when in conversation, which indicates that they understand what is being said (they are orientated), or do they appear to be distracted or preoccupied?
- Is the person's mood consistent with the interaction? For example, if in response to the question: *'Do you generally have a good appetite?'* the person laughs loudly as though being told the punchline of a joke, their response mood might be regarded as incongruent with the issues being discussed.

Where the person repeatedly struggles to answer, or seems to experience difficulty with questions, the mental health nurse might adapt their communication to avoid humiliating the person, so that they are not embarrassed or distressed. In these circumstances it may help for example to avoid the further use of closed questions but still address the *themes* of the assessment.

Other similar examples to the one above that might apply in different areas of mental health nursing include the following.

Example 2: a young adult male has been readmitted to an open acute mental health unit under a community treatment order (CTO) (Mental Health Act, 1983 reviewed 2007) after ceasing his prescribed antipsychotic medication and reportedly responding to auditory hallucinations. While waiting in the reception area he has been observed to be animatedly talking, laughing and smiling while no one else is present. He has no knowledge that he has been observed doing this.

Example 3: a middle-aged female has been referred by her GP due to low mood and depression. She is waiting in the reception area, averting eye contact and exhibiting a closed posture. She appears in an unkempt condition.

Q: What do you think might be the consistent learning points that we can take from these three examples?

A: *In all three cases certain aspects of the person's behaviour may lead us to form initial impressions about them. However, as opposed to drawing conclusions from this information it is better to regard it as a cue for further investigation, to be aware that these are only first impressions, and to seek additional information to prove or disprove our preconceptions.*

In order to implement an evidence-based approach to assessment, it is necessary to fully understand the person and their circumstances. Therefore, careful attention needs to be paid to how we understand and interpret a person's communication, and the mental health nurse also needs to make considered use of interpersonal skills.

Conclusion

Assessment is more than simply the collection of information but involves the effective use of communication and interpersonal skills to gain an accurate understanding of the person, and the way in which they are experiencing issues with their mental health. An approach focused solely on gathering facts will fail to reveal the subtle connections and nuances which are essential if we are to fully understand not only what the person is undergoing but also their view of the issues they are experiencing and what it means for them.

If the person feels at ease and that the assessor is genuinely interested in them then they are more likely to engage and the assessment will be a positive experience. This is important as there will be more than one assessment: it is an ongoing process.

In the initial assessment the service user is likely to feel anxious and this may mean they are less likely to engage. However, by remaining aware and adapting flexibly and therapeutically to the service user's feelings, by being conscious of how we present ourselves and how we communicate with the service user, we can begin to engage with them more effectively, create an effective therapeutic rapport and gain a clearer understanding of the problem(s) they are experiencing.

To conclude, here are some reflective questions for you to consider.

Q: What might be the benefits of an assessment in which the person has felt able to engage?

A: Often assessment provides the opportunity for people with mental health difficulties to talk about their problem(s). In some cases the person might not have anyone to confide in, or if they do, they may not be able to talk about their problem(s). In these circumstances the person might see their problems from a fresh perspective, or feel a sense of relief at having been able to tell someone else. Often by telling someone else the scale of the problem is reduced or made more manageable, or the person sees more hope and potential for positive progress. In this sense assessment performs a therapeutic function and the use of interpersonal and communication skills has an important role.

Q: Reflect on your practice experience. Have the assessments you have seen been affected by the person's being in a state of crisis? Think about the circumstances and how a given assessment might have been better planned.

Reference

Skinner, V. and Wrycraft, N. (2014) *CBT fundamentals: theory and cases*. Maidenhead: Open University Press.

Further reading

Bowers, L., Brennan, G., Winship, G. and Theodoridou, C. (2009) Talking with acutely psychotic people: communication skills for nurses and others spending time with people who are very mentally ill, www.iop.kcl.ac.uk/iopweb/blob/downloads/locator/l_436_Talking.pdf, accessed 9 December 2014.

Burnard, P. (2003) Ordinary chat and therapeutic conversation: phatic communication and mental health nursing, *Journal of Psychiatric and Mental Health Nursing*, 10: 678–82.

Bach, S. and Grant, A. (2011) *Communication and interpersonal skills in learning*, 2nd edn. Exeter: Learning Matters.

Crawford, P. and Brown, B. (2009) Mental health communication between service users and professionals: disseminating practice-congruent research, *Mental Health Review Journal*, 14(3): 31–9.

Hughes, C., Herron, S. and Younge, J. (2014) *CBT for mild to moderate depression: a guide to low intensity interventions*. Maidenhead: Open University Press.

Moore, E. (2014) What are interpersonal skills in nursing?, www.ehow.com/list_6605775_interpersonal-skills-nursing_.html, accessed 9 December 2014.

3 Engaging with the service user in assessment

Introduction

In the previous chapter we explored why it is important to be able to communicate effectively. By being able to use communication and interpersonal skills we are more likely to engage effectively with the service user. In this chapter we will expand on these ideas, and from engagement consider how we can then develop the therapeutic relationship.

Initiating and sustaining effective therapeutic relationships not only involves the active use of communication and interpersonal skills but also a genuine interest in and positive regard for the service user. This chapter begins by discussing an understanding of engagement, before looking at empathy. Next we consider aspects of verbal and non-verbal behaviour that contribute to forming a positive therapeutic rapport. Finally we discuss the importance of assertive communication in equal and mutually collaborative therapeutic relationships.

By the end of this chapter the reader will:

- understand a definition of engagement
- have considered the role of empathy
- be able to appreciate the importance of therapeutic rapport and assertiveness.

Engagement

For mental health nursing assessments to gain as complete and accurate picture of the issues that are relevant for the person as possible, it is necessary for them to be fully engaged in the process. With this in mind it is worth the mental health nurse carefully considering how they can adopt an approach that will maximize the opportunity for the service user to participate in the assessment.

Engagement refers to the mental health nurse and the person being assessed actively working together, establishing common ground and a shared understanding.

Unlike in other relationships that develop gradually, in assessment the person is often quickly expected to disclose personal and private information to another individual they might not have met before and hardly know.

Q: How do you think the person might feel in this situation?

A: There are many different answers but here are a few possibilities:
- the person may feel vulnerable about revealing deeply personal information to another person they do not know
- they may feel a sense of shame and embarrassment

(continued)

- *they may have very strong feelings about the issues being discussed*
- *they may not wish to talk about the problem through not wishing to think about something that they find distressing*
- *they may feel resentful and angry and view the assessor as a self-appointed 'expert'.*

At the heart of all meaningful relationships in life is trust. Therefore, in order to engage the person it is necessary for the mental health nurse to demonstrate qualities that might be worthy of the person feeling able to trust them.

Q: Think of a person that you trust in your life. Whether a relative, friend or colleague, what qualities do they have that make you feel you can trust them?

A: *It is likely that you identified a person that understands you, values you, believes in you or has your best interests at heart. Their qualities might include:*

- *a caring attitude*
- *discretion/confidentiality*
- *courage*
- *fairness*
- *good advice*
- *honesty*
- *integrity.*

When working with people with mental health issues, how we use our interpersonal skills will determine whether the person feels comfortable and able to engage with us and whether we are worthy of their trust. A prerequisite of being trustworthy is genuineness and authenticity, and this relates to more than the words that we use in conversation but also to how we act and what we do, and what we believe and the principles and values we hold.

The more our personal and professional values overlap the more authentic we will appear to the person with whom we are seeking to engage (see partnership working, Chapter 6). This is because our communication and responses will be genuine and natural, as opposed to artificial and contrived. However, it is still necessary to continually reflect, because we all have blind spots or preconceptions, and to continuously assimilate new learning into the beliefs we already hold.

Q: What practical actions might we carry out to facilitate a person's engagement?

A: *The simple actions that we might take include:*
- *actively involving the person in setting the agenda for the assessment*
- *regularly asking whether they are okay to continue*
- *checking back using the words that person has used to ensure that the meaning of what they have said can be understood*
- *demonstrating positive feedback for the person's achievements, positive capabilities and strengths*

(continued)

- *telling the person what assessment documentation is being completed and why*
- *at the end of the assessment summarizing what you understand are the issues that have been discussed along with the outcomes, and asking whether there is anything that you have missed*
- *avoiding making any comments which might seem judgemental.*

Most people would agree that a good basis for professional practice is to treat everyone equally and to fully engage with them wherever possible. Yet to understand how we carry this out as mental health nurses it is necessary to consciously reflect on our communication and to continuously learn and develop these skills (see reflection, Chapter 9).

Next we will build on this understanding and consider the crucial role that is performed by empathy.

The role of empathy

A central quality that mental health nurses require to be able to engage with people is **empathy**. Empathy means putting ourselves 'in the other person's shoes' and trying to understand how that person might feel. Yet as we are not actually in their situation, while we might try to understand, we can never totally appreciate their perspective. The best we can ever achieve is to approximate what it might be like. Despite this, adopting an empathic approach is extremely helpful in seeing how the world appears to the other person. Using an empathic approach involves suspending our own views, judgements and interpretations and instead trying to understand the other person's viewpoint, and why they might think how they do in the circumstances.

Q: How might we begin to develop an empathic approach?

A: *We could ask ourselves, how does the person perceive their current circumstances and immediate situation? We might not have made the same choices, or acted in the same way, but this will help us understand the person and form a better rapport with them if we can appreciate their reasoning.*

It is important to look at the major challenges that have occurred in the person's life, both in the recent and more distant past and to understand how they responded. They may have coped very well over a prolonged period of time under extreme difficulties, and only recently experienced problems due to the challenges finally exceeding their coping mechanisms. Alternatively, they may have experienced major difficulties but do not feel that these have had a major influence. In some cases the person may say they are unaffected but you may feel that they clearly are. Or it may be that there is no real explanation from the person's life events to account for their current mental health issue(s).

Rogers (1951) suggests that in order to ensure that the therapeutic alliance is effective, the mental health nurse ought to have – in addition to empathy – warmth, genuineness and unconditional positive regard for the person. As we are all human, and shaped by many different influences and experiences, we need to reflect upon and challenge our preconceptions, so that these do not hinder the development of therapeutic rapport.

Yet in order to actively use empathy it is necessary to convey this understanding *back* to the service user. This will be evident through interpersonal and non-verbal communication – for example, eye contact, facial expressions, gestures, verbal feedback and comments – that are congruent with the service user's and show that their feelings and views have been heard and understood. Empathy may also be evident through verbal feedback and comments.

Q: Which of the comments below made by a mental health nurse to a service user effectively express empathic feelings, and which are inappropriate? Consider the reasons for your choices, and then see if they match the answers below:

1 'I understand how you might feel like that'
2 'I know exactly how you feel'
3 'I can see how in that situation you felt how you did'
4 'What you should have done is...'

A: Answers 1 and 3 are empathic, as the mental health nurse is not necessarily suggesting that they would have acted in the same way and is not claiming to understand exactly how the service user feels. Answer 2 is mistaken, as the mental health nurse claims to know exactly how the service user feels, which is not possible, as while their life experiences may be similar or comparable they are not the same, and so this is a false claim. Answer 4 is also incorrect, as the mental health nurse is telling the service user what they ought to have done, which could represent judging the service user. Also, this answer does not really demonstrate a commitment to listening to the person, or valuing their experience.

When seeking to empathize with a service user we may become aware of our own preconceptions. For example, I am due to carry out an assessment on a person who has previously committed a violent offence. Due to knowledge of the person's past I may behave in a more subdued and less engaging manner in the assessment, at times avoiding eye contact and asking fewer questions than usual, with the result that I engage less well with the person than I might with other people. On reflection I may feel that I was affected by what I knew about the person. Though the difference in behaviour might only be slight, my negative view of the person influenced my actions and behaviour and how I engaged with them, and hence the effectiveness of the assessment.

However, preconceptions can also have the reverse effect. For example, in carrying out an assessment of an older man with dementia I read in the case notes that there is a long history of domestic violence towards his wife preceding the man's experiencing dementia. After the assessment a colleague who jointly carried out the assessment with me praised my perseverance in persisting and being positive and upbeat, in spite of the man's persistently negative responses. On reflection I felt that I did not achieve an effective therapeutic rapport due to the lack of congruence between me and the service user, and even that my persistent positivity 'wound him up' and I overcompensated in a way that I might not have normally in trying not to make my negative feelings evident. Our preconceptions can lead us to compensate in order to make up for our negative feelings.

It is possible to become very concerned and focused on the influence of our pre-conceptions on others or to believe that our perceptions about a situation, either positive or negative, predispose the outcome of an assessment.

Q: What advice might we give to the person for whom this is the case?

A: Working in situations where our values are challenged can often feel uncomfortable. However, it is a central part of responsible and professional practice to share concerns where these occur, and to work towards constructive and professional solutions. Sources of support include:

- mentors
- clinical supervision
- colleagues and peer support
- line managers.

It is important to remember that everyone has preconceptions and prejudices. However, it is healthy to explore and discuss these and continue to develop our values and attitudes towards others (NMC, 2015).

Q: Think of a mental health issue which you find hard to understand or relate to. Now consider what has influenced your understanding.

A: A possible answer might be: 'It is difficult for me to understand how a person might feel a desire to carry out self-harm. When hearing about the ways in which people have harmed themselves I struggle to think how I would feel in that situation, because I just cannot relate to having thoughts that might rationalize that choice of action, or how it might realistically feel to contemplate or prepare to carry out self-harm.

'In reflecting on this I realize I have a very strong aversion to pain, and believe I have a low pain threshold. Also, while I have known people that have carried out self-harm, I have never really had any exposure to it, and so while I do not feel a sense of judging this behaviour I feel more of a sense of guilt that I cannot relate to it and cannot really understand it.'

Q: Now consider an area of mental health, a mental health problem, or a behaviour that is often displayed by a particular client group that you find hard to understand. Reflect on the nature of your feelings, and why you feel them, and actions you might take to address these issues.

It may be you related to the above comments and that you do find self-harming hard to understand. The same may apply for any number of mental health issues from anorexia to substance misuse. The breadth of issues that are incorporated within mental health, and the range of different factors involved, mean that we cannot possibly relate to everything and everyone we might encounter. However, it is important to be aware of how we feel, as this may exert an effect on how we relate to, and engage with, service users.

Q: Now think of a mental health issue that you feel a sense of understanding towards. Again, think about what has influenced this perception.

A: A possible answer might be: 'I noticed when working with a service user that I feel a sense of identification with people that experience depression, and can understand how everything feels like an effort, that sometimes things seem to go slowly, and it is hard to concentrate on anything. Also, sometimes I am comfortable with the silences and delays when conversing with the person.

'In reflecting on this, I realize it may be influenced by my background. I grew up with close contact with a relative who experienced recurrent bouts of depression and understood how it was for them.'

Often empathy is derived from our life experience. In this sense there is a felt understanding that can be extremely meaningful. However, it is still worth remembering that everyone's experience is different and while we might undergo the same events, how we feel about them and recall them may differ. It is important to be open to feelings of identification, but it is also necessary to question what they mean for us, as they can lead to positive or negative preconceptions. For example, a mental health nurse may have grown up with a parent who experienced depression and found that their otherwise loving, communicative and caring parent became self-absorbed, preoccupied and distant for periods of time when depressed. The mental health nurse may feel that they have a good understanding of depression and believe that they relate well to people with depression. Yet they find that they feel negative and uncomfortable when working with people experiencing depression.

Alternatively, it is possible to feel a sense of affinity towards people with certain mental health issues through this kind of life experience, and be able to relate to them seemingly intuitively, which eases the engagement process. In the best functioning therapeutic relationships there is a shared sense of knowing and understanding. In the final part of this chapter we will consider such therapeutic rapport.

Therapeutic rapport and assertiveness

Rapport is the development of a harmonious and trusting understanding with another person and can be established through the use of communication techniques. Rapport is the common ground or content of engagement and includes: active listening, turn-taking, demonstrating an interest in the person and their story, and offering feedback.

Listening is a surprisingly active process, yet if carried out effectively it success-fully encourages the person to impart more information (Hughes et al., 2014).

Q: Consider and then write down the methods we use to demonstrate to others that we are actively listening to them.

A: We demonstrate listening by our verbal gestures in response to what a person is say-ing. These can validate what they are saying but can also encourage the person to say more. For example, comments such as: '...that must have been difficult...' in response to a problem or bad experience. We also ask questions about what the person has said and seek clarification – for example: '...and then what did you do?' Or '...how did that make you feel?' We summarize what the person has said in order to check that our understanding is correct: 'If I understand you correctly what you have told me is...'. Our facial responses and expressions encourage the person to communicate more freely and demonstrate our enthusiasm and interest, or that we share the emotion the person is describing.

However, all of these responses need to be genuine in terms of being realistic, and authentic. Communication which is exaggerated or artificial can have a damaging effect and stifle a developing rapport.

Turn-taking in discussion is subtle and norms vary depending on culture, the nature of the encounter and the type of conversation. For example, you might know a person but then speak on the phone to them and experience a previously unen-countered difficulty of knowing when to speak without interrupting one another or of there being lengthy silences. The absence of visual cues and non-verbal gestures can often undermine a previously effortless relationship. In mental health settings the service user may be distressed, anxious or distracted and the assessment may benefit from the mental health nurse actively facilitating turn-taking in conversation, which can enhance rapport and develop trust. The therapeutic relationship may ben-efit from the mental health nurse speaking less and encouraging the service user to speak and participate in the conversation as much as possible.

Interest in the person is important. Assessment involves establishing a coher-ent picture of the person and their situation. Rarely is everything that we need to know about the person readily available or volunteered. Instead, it is usually neces-sary to consider the *gaps* in our understanding of the person's situation and then find out more. It is necessary to demonstrate interest in the person by thinking about what they have experienced, who they are and what makes them that person, and to ask questions to clarify their perspective of events. We may need to ask about their values, motivations and beliefs, or seek clarification if these are not already self-evident, or are only partially understood.

It is important to give **feedback** to the person in order to demonstrate that we have heard and understood what has been said – not only in terms of the *content* of what has been said (although this is a benefit of providing feedback) but also in terms of the feelings and meanings that are *attached* to what is said in order to pro-vide acknowledgement of the person's feelings and reactions.

Feedback needs to be genuine and honest. For example, if the person is distressed but I cannot understand why, then I might respond by acknowledging the extent of their distress: *'I see that this made you very upset'*. On the other hand, if I can understand why the person is distressed, I might say: *'I can see why this might make you upset'*. However, it is important to reflect on striking the right balance in providing feedback. For example, if the person is describing an experience that I too have had, it is necessary to avoid burdening them with my feelings. Alternatively, if I cannot understand how the person could be upset over a certain issue it is not helpful for me to trivialize their concern to avoid imposing my own preconceptions. If there is to be effective engagement, then each person needs to feel empowered.

Assertiveness refers to both parties having an equal role and influence in the relationship. When seeking to develop engagement, relationships often require negotiation. Here are some examples.

When assessing a person who is self-critical, how do we encourage assertiveness? The person might say: *'We went bowling, and as usual I wasn't very good at it'*. If the assessor challenges this statement they then reinforce the person's low self-esteem and appear to be in the role of the expert, which undermines the power balance in the relationship.

Rather than making a specific comment on the person's statement, acknowledging you have heard what they have said may be the best course of action. If there are other instances of self-criticism during the conversation, it may be possible to later reflect to the person that they at times seem to be harsh on themselves. Where this is a repeated pattern it might be helpful to encourage the person to reflect on their self-criticism and, for example, ask them: *'What would you say to a friend who said that to you?'*

On other occasions the mental health nurse will need to 'claim power', in order to exercise an equal role in the assessment. For example, Chris has been detained under Section 2 of the Mental Health Act. He is very intelligent and articulate but extremely angry about needing to remain on the mental health unit. He feels that everyone is against him and has consistently been rude to other service users and the ward staff. Tina, who is his key worker for the afternoon, is newly qualified and feels quite nervous about working with Chris as well as being intimidated by him. However, she approaches Chris at the beginning of the shift to ask whether he would like to have a one-to-one. Chris talks aggressively to Tina: *'Look at your posture, standing there with your arms folded – don't you know that's closed body posture? Don't they teach you anything at uni?'* Tina unfolds her arms and adopts a more open body posture. She feels embarrassed by Chris's comment but then says in an even tone: *'Listen Chris, I know you're annoyed but perhaps talking about it might help?'*

Q: What did Tina do right in this situation?

A: Tina communicated in a manner that understood the reason for Chris being upset. Her comment focused on Chris's need and sought to offer a constructive outcome to his situation, rather than responding to her sense of embarrassment or awkwardness, and therefore established a balance in power in the relationship.

Conclusion

In this chapter we discussed engagement, before moving on to consider the important contribution that empathy makes in developing an effective and genuine therapeutic rapport with the person. Next we looked at a number of elements that are evident within and contribute towards an effective therapeutic rapport.

Within assessments, the techniques that we use will necessarily differ. However there are frequently occurring skills that lead to success and these can be acquired and developed with practice and experience. Yet to acquire real meaning, these skills and techniques need to be supported by values and principles, and always being truthful and open is essential even though it can at times be challenging. As we change as people it is important to continually reflect on our values and views, and be honest with ourselves regarding the empathy we feel towards the service users that we assess. For more on values, see the last section of Chapter 1.

In all assessments that we carry out in specialist mental health services it is necessary to consider risk. Therefore in the next chapter we will consider this topic in terms of what risk is, and how we understand and manage it.

References

Hughes, C., Herron, S. and Younge, J. (2014) *CBT for mild to moderate depression: a guide to low intensity intervention*. Maidenhead: Open University Press.

NMC (Nursing and Midwifery Council) (2015) *The code: professional standards of practice and behaviour for nurses and midwives*. London: NMC, www.nmc-uk.org, accessed 30 January, 2015.

Rogers, C. (1951) *Client-centered therapy*. Cambridge, MA: The Riverside Press.

Further reading

Bach, S. and Grant, A. (2011) *Communication and interpersonal skills in learning*, 2nd edn. Exeter: Learning Matters.

Crawford, P. and Brown, B. (2009) Mental health communication between service users and professionals: disseminating practice-congruent research, *Mental Health Review Journal*, 14(3): 31–9.

Department of Health (DoH) (2006) *Best practice competencies and capabilities for pre-registration mental health nurses in England: the Chief Nursing Officer's review of mental health nursing*, http://hsc.uwe.ac.uk/net/mentor/Data/Sites/1/GalleryImages/Nursing/Best%20practice%20and%20 competencies%20and%20capabilities%20for%20pre-reg%20mental%20health%20nurses%20in%20 England.pdf, accessed 9 December 2014.

Mills, H. and Dombeck, M. (2005) Resilience, compassion and empathy, www.mentalhelp.net/poc/ view_doc.php?type=doc&id=5796&cn=298, accessed 9 December 2014.

4 Risk assessment

Introduction

An expectation of any mental health nursing assessment is for there to be a clear and considered assessment of the risks that the person presents and to which they are vulnerable. This is with good reason, as assessments often occur in crisis situations, where there is a very real element of risk. In working with risk it is necessary to be able to strike a balance between being adaptable to individual situations and circumstances, yet also to identify where commonly evident risks may be apparent.

In this chapter we begin with a definition of risk and the range of features this covers, before looking at approaches and issues to consider in risk assessment and then at measures in risk management.

By the end of the chapter the reader will:

- understand how we define risk and risk assessment
- have considered approaches to risk assessment
- appreciate approaches to risk management.

A definition and understanding of risk

In the situations where mental health nursing assessments are carried out we are often working with people whose actions are uncertain, who may represent risk in various forms, or be at risk from others. Risk is also often described as being dynamic, in that the nature and form that it takes can quickly change to produce new challenges or concerns. Therefore, assessment requires very careful consideration of how and in what forms risk is both evident and potential.

Risk can be understood as the likelihood or probability of an event occurring that is generally untoward but can also be positive (see Chapter 7, p. 54). **Risk assessment** in mental health nursing is the process through which mental health nurses identify the probability of an event occurring that has potentially harmful consequences.

Q: How do mental health nurses approach risk assessments?

A: It is rare for an event with untoward or unfortunate circumstances to occur completely without any predisposing circumstances. Even impulsive or unpredictable behaviours require triggers or a combination of predisposing circumstances to be in place that if we were aware of them might permit the situation to be avoided, or the impact(s) of the effect(s) to be reduced. Although it can't be totally eliminated, it is still possible that we can know something about a person's propensity to risk and put plans in place to reduce the likelihood of harmful effects.

Risk assessments involve a detailed consideration of the person and their circumstances, based on what is known, as opposed to opinions or preconceptions. Consistent with assessment being a two-stage process (see Chapter 1, p. 6), it is necessary to gather all of the relevant facts and information before forming a conclusion. Assessing risk permits the mental health nurse to consider in what areas the person may represent a risk, or be at risk, and to then plan accordingly.

The best source of information is the person in terms of what is important to them and the reasons for their behaviour. But in some cases – for example, a person who loses control and becomes violent towards others – the behaviour may not be explicable. Alternatively, in the case of a person experiencing dementia, for example, they may not be aware of the risks.

Such information can be gathered from:

- previous casenotes
- observing the person and their emerging patterns of behaviour
- what we learn from other nurses in the team
- other professionals involved in the person's care
- the person's family, carers and significant others.

Q: What range of behaviours does risk include?

A: You may have thought of the following:

- self-harm
- suicide
- violence or aggression to, or from, others
- self-neglect
- risk of exploiting others (emotional, financial, psychological, sexual)
- vulnerability to exploitation by others (emotional, financial, psychological, sexual).

The aspects of risk highlighted above have significantly differing features and in practice specific assessment tools are used in their assessment. In this chapter we will be discussing generic assessments of risk that the assessor is more likely to notice and therefore the examples provided are of an immediate or crisis-led nature, such as violence, aggression to others or suicide. Other risks that may be less clearly apparent may be equally as debilitating yet more particular or less obvious. For example, risk of financial, emotional or sexual exploitation to which the service user is prone or might carry out.

Often several factors combine that contribute to the risk. For example, a person may be experiencing the distressing effects of mental illness, misusing substances and also experiencing or have experienced exploitation or abuse by another person. These factors may act to influence one another, or be mutually interdependent and reinforce one another. The settings where mental health nurses frequently encounter service users can also exacerbate the situation. For example, being admitted to an acute inpatient unit can be an uncertain, anxiety-provoking and upsetting time for a person and may escalate factors contributing to their risk profile.

Q: What information should a risk assessment include?

A: You may have thought of the following:
- an accurate, succinct and clear explanation of the specific nature of the risks that the person might represent, or to which they may be vulnerable
- the circumstances, environment or triggers that may make the risky behaviour more likely to occur
- whether the risk has any individualistic or specific characteristics, for example whether it could occur suddenly if the person is prone to acting impetuously, or through a specific medium if a person uses a certain object as a weapon
- the possible severity of harm occurring as a result of the risk event.

A risk assessment should:

- be up to date and regularly reviewed
- be rigorous and detailed
- offer clear guidance concerning risk
- provide guidance on risk minimization
- include a risk management plan.

Approaches to risk assessment

Risk assessments occur in a variety of environments from the community to inpatient settings. However, the environment ought not to dictate the nature of the risk assessment, or be used casually. For example, inpatient areas provide greater resources for directly reducing risk through enabling the service user to be observed, and their whereabouts and actions monitored, and a safe and secure environment is created as a result. Although all of this may be necessary for some service users, it ought to be predicated based on an individual risk assessment, and rationales for each intervention, as opposed to routinely being imposed for all service users in this setting.

However, situations can rapidly change. Effective risk assessment requires careful and astute understanding of specific situations, and an appreciation of how the person responds in different situations. For example, there may be patterns of certain types of behaviour, or situations where particular responses are triggered. Assessment tools for specific risks are available and some aspects of risk – for example vulnerability to emotional or psychological abuse, or exploitation – may be less easy to detect or measure than some other risks. However, there are some consistent principles that offer a reliable and schematic approach to the assessment of any risk.

Q: What aspects might we consider in a generalized risk assessment?

A: *The following elements are useful to consider:*

What happens in the risk event? *For example, the person has carried out self-harm by cutting their arm. A factual description of the event might not seem to summarize what has occurred but will help us to reflect on the event and assist in removing the subjective effect of feelings.*

The factors that are active in the risk:

- *Where did the event happen?*
- *Who is there?*
- *What tools, materials or other resources are involved or used in the risk event?*

What does the behaviour mean to the person? *What intention does the person have in carrying out the behaviour?*

In the case of a person who has self-harmed by cutting, applying each of these factors, they may have:

- been in their bedroom on an inpatient unit
- been alone
- used a razor blade they had carefully hidden from the ward staff and other service users
- felt a sense of relief and release from tension or were able to experience some form of feeling, compared with their usual sense of numbness.

In this situation we are considering a specific event, or occurrence. However to assess risk more comprehensively, it is useful to assess a wide range of information and to consider events that have previously occurred as well as the situation in the present. Different risks will require an emphasis or focus on certain phenomena. However, an overall framework within which all risks might be considered includes: demographic factors, background history, clinical history, physical factors, psychological factors and the current context (Wellman, 2006; Noonan, 2013), and these categories are outlined in more detail below:

Demographic factors

- age
- gender
- ethnicity.

Background factors

- significant life events
- family
- friends and social network
- education
- previous employment history
- where the person lives
- financial issues.

Clinical profile

- previous mental health history
- diagnoses
- whether the person has engaged with care
- how the person feels about their diagnosis.

Physical health

- current physical health status
- previous physical health issues
- whether the physical health issues are effectively managed.

Psychological factors

- mood
- motivation: does the person feel hopeless about their life? Are they prone to impulsive actions? Do they feel worthless or that their life lacks value or meaning?

Current context

- the circumstances that have led to the person's current episode of mental ill-health.

The person's perspective

- How do they perceive their risk profile and overall situation?

In summary, we have considered a variety of factors that may be evident in risk assessment. These cover a wide range of the person's bio-psychosocial functioning, and some will feature more or less prominently than others. Yet often risk is like a stone being dropped into a pool of water, creating ripples that emanate far from the source. Therefore in assessment it is always worth reflecting on the scope and extent to which risk is active and to form an in-depth understanding of the person and their perception of the world.

Risk management

Risk management is the introduction of measures that effectively address the issues in relation to which the person has been assessed as vulnerable. It is worth remembering that although risk management reduces the possibility of untoward events happening due the nature of these phenomena as changeable, we can never entirely eliminate risk.

Q: How can we identify effective risk management measures?

A: *Risk management relies upon:*

* *Appreciating the often complex and interconnected range of issues contributing to the person's propensity for risk and understanding how these all act together. For example, the person may be low in mood, living alone, misusing substances and feeling as though they have lost all hope in life. The risk is created by the combination of factors leading to, for example, a significant deterioration in mood, self-neglect with the potential for harm to the person's physical health, or self-harming behaviour. Risk reduction will be achieved by addressing these factors.*
* *Understanding the person's perspective. How do they perceive their risks? Has the person developed a plan to end their life? Has the person acted impulsively at previous times in their life through not feeling able to handle their emotions in other ways?*
* *Identifying patterns and triggers. Are a certain set of circumstances in place at the time that the risk event occurs? For example, does the person self-harm after arguments with their partner about money?*
* *The expertise of the multidisciplinary team. Decisions regarding risk need to be as a result of discussion between the professionals involved in delivering care.*
* *What works with the person? Previous strategies that were successful for the person – for example, using distraction in the event of the person experiencing negative or distressing thoughts that trigger self-harming behaviour.*

It is important when considering these factors that the risk assessment does not become a process of collecting negative data about the person or a defensive exercise. Instead, previous risks or behaviour need to be seen in the context of the person's *present* circumstances. This will help to discover what has changed about the person's situation in comparison with previous similar instances when they were assessed. Viewing risk in this manner allows for the appreciation of differences or variations in the person's risk profile. All of these factors feed into an effective and comprehensive risk management plan that will meet the person's needs.

* Risk management aims to empower the person and encourage them to take responsibility for the risk. For example, agreeing with the person that in the event of their feeling the need to self-harm they should advise the ward staff.
* Risk management may also feed into other aspects of the person's care plan. For example, in care planning you can agree with the person who is on the inpatient unit certain dangers and necessary measures – for example, if there are concerns about their propensity to abscond this can be discussed and it can be agreed that in the event of their attempting to do so that it may be necessary to increase the level of observation. However, care should be taken to avoid such measures appearing to be punitive or coercive, as this only ensures concordance without working collaboratively with the person.

Conclusion

In this chapter we have examined risk and risk assessment, but also the range of behaviours that this includes and what ought to be included in a risk assessment. We next looked at approaches to risk assessment from a variety of perspectives and in relation to a range of factors before moving on to consider risk management.

Risk assessment is extremely important and a central component of a comprehensive assessment. Although it can be reduced, the dynamic nature of risk and the variable circumstances in which mental health nursing is carried out mean that risk can never be totally eradicated. However, it can be minimized. Within assessment it is important that all considerations of risk weigh up the relevant facts and consider predisposing factors, and that all observations and decisions are clearly based on evidence and can be justified. Through practice and experience, skills in risk assessment can be honed and developed. We next move on to look at care planning.

References

Noonan, I. (2013) Assessing and managing the risk of self-harm and suicide, in I. Norman and I. Ryrie (eds) *The art and science of mental health nursing: principles and practice*, 3rd edn. Maidenhead: Open University Press.

Wellman, N. (2006) Assessing risk, in C. Gamble and G. Brennan (eds) *Working with serious mental illness*, 2nd edn, pp. 145–64. London: Elsevier.

Further reading

Langan, J. and Lindow, V. (2004) Mental health service users and their involvement in risk assessment and management, www.jrf.org.uk/sites/files/jrf/414.pdf, accessed 9 December 2014.

Petch, E. (2001) Risk management in UK mental health services: an overvalued idea?, http://pb.rcpsych.org/content/25/6/203.full.pdf+html, accessed 9 December 2014.

5 Care planning

Introduction

Planning care requires skill in identifying and prioritizing needs and experience in practice and reflection on the part of the mental health nurse. Furthermore, in order to generate meaningful change and be effective for the service user, it is essential to collaboratively involve them in partnership through discussing, negotiating and agreeing the care plan.

In this chapter we will discuss a definition and understanding of what care planning is, before looking at approaches to the planning of care, and then consider the strategies we might use to do this.

By the end of this chapter the reader will be able to:

- define what a care plan and care planning are
- understand how to approach the planning of care
- consider communication techniques in care planning.

A definition and understanding of care planning

Care plans are measures to address the person's mental health needs that are developed from assessment. A **care plan** is a description of the interventions and actions that will occur in the person's care; an outline of the desired outcome(s) against which progress is measured; and a record of the agreement of the service user and mental health nurse, along with the date for review of each care intervention.

Individual needs are likely to have particular care plans focused on specific issues, whereby a number of interventions are all focused on achieving the overall outcome. Therefore the person's overall care plan may well be comprised of several individualized and need-specific care plans, as demonstrated in the case studies in Section 3 of this book.

A care plan can take many forms, ranging from a letter to casenotes to a discharge summary, however increasingly they are computerized and in a standardized format.

Q: Can you think of the advantages and disadvantages of a computerized care plan?

A: Some possible answers might be:

- Advantage: a computerized care plan with standard headings is easy to access, and will contain the same range of information for everyone.
- Disadvantages: over time staff may become complacent and write the same information under each heading, and not use their initiative. This may lead to care not being personalized and service users not feeling that their needs are being recognized. Therefore if computerized care plans with standard headings are used, it may help to add suggestions under these of possibilities of what the interventions and actions might be to promote innovative thinking and person-centred care planning.

Often a care plan will begin by providing a brief biography of the service user and then summarize the service user's range of needs, followed by the focused plans that address different and specific requirements. The design of the care plan may vary, however there is generally:

- a problem statement
- intervention
- outcome
- date of review and the signatures of the mental health nurse and service user.

These criteria are discussed in more detail in Chapter 7 but represent a logical, coherent and chronological structure, through which care can be assessed, planned, delivered and evaluated.

Q: Think about why we plan care. Write down your answers and then read those below to see whether there are any that you missed.

A: Mental health nurses plan care:

- to move the service user's care forward and promote their recovery
- to set clear and achievable goals, against which progress can later be measured
- to organize the service user's care, as often there are multiple care plans and areas of need
- to communicate and provide clear guidance to the people delivering the care, as often there are multiple professionals, agencies or carers involved who all need to know about the person's care plan
- to actively use evidence in informing the service user's care
- to work in accordance with the law and the requirements of the Nursing and Midwifery Council (NMC) (2015), other healthcare regulatory professional bodies and local trust policy and guidance.

In **care planning** there is a process of deliberation, negotiation and discussion of the information that has been gathered during assessment, and the measures at our disposal and within our resources that might be useful for the service user to aid their recovery. In order for meaningful care planning to occur it is important that this process occurs, as active collaboration and involvement of the service user in developing the care plan is essential to form a meaningful and personalized plan.

This involves several stages, as shown in Figure 5.1.

Discussion of the range of options that are available between the mental health nurse and the service user
Negotiation and comparing view points of the service user and mental health nurse regarding mutual priorities and the preferred measures to include in the care plan
Agreement and decisions over what are the prioritized measures, and the rationales supporting the choice of interventions. Who is to carry out which actions and when
Making a commitment to carry out the plan and agreeing timeframes for action
Signing and dating the care plan

Figure 5.1 The stages of care planning

Care planning is a process in itself and not simply an extension of assessment, and the measures that will be used need to be developed and discussed with the service user. Therefore the engagement and therapeutic rapport established with the service user, as discussed in Chapters 2 and 3, is developed further. There needs to be time allowed for reflection on the issues and the preferred interventions or actions that will be chosen. In addition to this, other members of the multidisciplinary team may need to be involved in order to access their specialist skills and knowledge in contributing to the plan, or as a possible direct referral for therapeutic input or assessment as a care planned measure. Furthermore, within the bounds of confidentiality, carers or significant others of the service user may be consulted, especially if they are to be directly involved in delivering care.

Approaches to planning care

It is often the case in practice that every need that the service user has is care planned and numerous interventions identified, with the consequence that the overall care plan represents a wish list that can never be achieved. Sometimes this arises from a desire not to overlook any area of need. However, it does not represent effective care planning skills. Instead it is preferable to agree fewer interventions but choose those that are of a more pressing need and of greater importance. This involves greater skill and expertise on the part of the mental health nurse, in terms of clinical knowledge in distinguishing between wants and needs, and also involves good communication and interpersonal skills in collaborating in an effective partnership with the service user to negotiate and balance clinical priorities with the service user's preferences.

Q: What do you think is the difference between a want and a need? At the top of a piece of paper, halfway in from the left-hand side, write the word 'wants'. Then in the middle of the piece of paper draw a vertical line. Next, at the top of the right-hand side write the word 'needs'. Then write down activities of living that fit under each of these headings. What consistent features do you notice about your wants? What is consistent concerning your needs? What is the difference?

A: A need is an item or resource that we all require. At the most basic level we need air, water, food, shelter and an environment that is temperate and safe. Not having access to these threatens not only continued good physical and mental health but also life. In contrast, a want is something that I may like but which I can continue to live and maintain physical and mental health without. Abraham Maslow developed a 'hierarchy of human needs' which consists of a pyramid with different needs situated on the various ascending layers, ranging from those that we need simply to survive, to those that we might wish for, such as loving relationships and feeling valued (Cherry, 2015).

In mental health the distinction between needs and wants is less obvious. Many would argue that social contact with others is a basic psychological human need, and the absence of this can lead to detrimental consequences for mental and even physical health. For example, if I am an older person living alone with restricted mobility and rarely see other people then I may regard my radio or television as my main source of social contact and company and therefore these items may become necessities as opposed to things I simply want.

How people make decisions about their personal wants and needs is highly subjective, especially for people with mental health issues. Understanding the individual's perceptions of wants and needs is crucial to working with them to form a care plan.

Example 1: Thomas has obsessive compulsive disorder and spends his days walking a specific route in his local area, leaving his house very early in the morning and returning in the evening. He collects what seem to be random items but which he specifically selects and stores at his home which has become filled with such objects so that he can only access his bed by climbing over things. The local council's environmental health department have served him with a notice to clean up the house, or this will be carried out for him. Thomas is very upset and feels embarrassed and guilty about his behaviour but is fearful of the loss of his collection. He blames himself for the state of his house but feels unable to resist the urges to collect items or deviate from his ritualized behaviour.

Example 2: Alice lives in a council-owned flat. Her rent is paid for by housing benefit but Alice believes there is a plot to evict her from the flat and so pays her rent in full each week. To avoid problems at the council offices where Alice pays the money, her social worker has arranged for the council to accept the money but pay it into

Alice's bank account. Despite having substantial savings, Alice refuses to take any of the money out of her bank. She avoids other people and her only company is her dog. She feeds him the most expensive dog food that she can buy and regularly takes him to the vet for health checks. However Alice often goes without food and does not switch the heating on for fear of acquiring debts.

How we perceive and provide for our wants and needs varies and we can only understand the rationales for these decisions by asking the service user about their viewpoint and perspective. Often people overlook their personal needs and this can have consequences for their longer-term mental and physical health and well-being. People with mental health issues also often lack social contacts and friendship networks that act as protective factors against mental illness. It is often the case that service users are not in employment, which can lead to or compound social exclusion and contribute to financial hardship, which in turn can detrimentally affect mental health. Therefore, when identifying care-planned interventions it is important that these are realistic and within the person's economic, psychological and social range of capability.

Techniques for communicating in care planning

Often it is the case that service users are reluctant to engage with mental health services. This can be for a variety of different reasons, and in some instances the person's mental health may directly present an obstacle – for example, the person may have strong feelings of paranoia which then involve mental health services. Other factors might include:

- low mood that may lead to a lack of motivation and self-esteem, and the service user not feeling able to, or confident of, achieving goals or making a change in their life
- the service user may be in a secure setting with limited opportunities for independent choices
- they may be in an inpatient care setting for a prolonged period of time, and feel there is very limited scope for autonomy or hope for recovery
- some service users also have negative feelings towards mental health services, associating them with becoming unwell and distressing experiences
- in other cases the service user may perceive having received, or have actually received, poor care that did not take account of their perspective or meet their needs
- some people value their independence and are reluctant to seek or accept help, even when they need it – they regard help as an interference
- negative portrayals of mental health services in the media leading to service users being reluctant to engage or having negative expectations.

The level of motivation and readiness for change that a person has is pivotal in working together to plan care, and in mental health can often be seen as a barrier (for further reading see Prochaska and DiClemente's 1984 transtheoretical stages of change model).

Q: Consider how you might communicate with a service user in planning their care in some of the above circumstances. Write down your answer(s) and then read the suggestion below. Compare the two.

A: A possible answer might be that it is necessary to understand the reason for the person being reluctant to engage with services. It is important to regard this as part of and incorporated into the process, as opposed to representing an inconvenient delay and an additional obstacle. Displaying empathy helps to appreciate the other person's perspective (see Chapter 3). Through understanding the reasons for the service user's reluctance to engage, we will form a more compatible rapport with them and perhaps identify solutions that fit the individual's specific need(s). We can do this by spending time and actively listening to the service user's concerns which demonstrates respect for their perspective and an interest in them (as also discussed in Chapter 3). It is important not to rush the service user – bear in mind that interviews, for example, have a limited duration, and an initial assessment may be a 'one off'. Instead, it helps to be flexible and it may therefore be necessary to meet the service user on several occasions to give them the time to discuss issues at their own pace. Positive regard, commitment and belief in the service user will also be demonstrated by drawing attention to their strengths and achievements, even if these are small. For example, if in the discussion the service user has engaged more than previously, remarking on this offers feedback that acknowledges progress. Reflecting before and after meetings with the service user on our own views as practitioners about the person and their care will help to reduce the influence of preconceptions about the service user.

The trust necessary for a therapeutic relationship can also often be developed by the mental health nurse carrying out actions demonstrating commitment and being reliable and consistent in accordance with principles and values. These include:

- being reliable in terms of always attending meetings on time, not cancelling appointments, following up on issues that we say we will and making a point of always remembering and recalling what has so far been discussed
- taking time to explain interventions in terms that make sense to the person
- fairly and objectively presenting the alternatives and choices that are available in the care options, to permit the person to make their own decisions on an informed basis
- explaining the importance of the service user participating in the planning of their care and that this is not just a beurocratic exercise
- allowing the person the opportunity to consider different care options
- being available at other times to discuss the person's concerns or reservations.

It is also helpful to:

- meet with the person individually before multidisciplinary meetings, care programme approach (CPA) meetings, ward rounds or reviews of care to avoid their feeling daunted by meeting with numerous professionals and feeling obliged to make quick decisions or to please others

- act as an advocate on behalf of the person during multidisciplinary meetings, CPA meetings, ward rounds or reviews of care to ensure their view is represented
- be willing to change or amend care plans depending upon the person's preferences and wishes so that the plans are a current and accurate reflection of practice
- ensure that care plans are written using the same language that the service user might use
- access clinical supervision or peer support to ensure that we are working accountably and responsibly, to our optimum level and to gain other perspectives and ideas.

Conclusion

In this chapter we have considered what a care plan is and the care planning process. We then looked at approaches that we might use in planning care with the service user before considering communication techniques that are useful. Within mental health there is often a reluctance on the part of the service user to participate in their care for a variety of different reasons. If we are to work effectively with the person it is important to have patience and seek to understand the service user's viewpoint, and to regard this as part of the process, rather than an inconvenience. The planning of care is an independent process in its own right following assessment, and provides a further opportunity to develop the collaborative relationship with the service user. We will now move on to consider the importance of partnership working and how to do this as part of assessment.

References

Cherry, K. (2015) Hierarchy of needs, http://psychology.about.com/od/theoriesofpersonality/a/hierarchyneeds.htm, accessed 17 April 2015.

Nursing and Midwifery Council (NMC) (2015) *The Code: Professional Standards of Practice and Behaviour for Nurses and Midwives.* London: NMC.

Prochaska, J.O. and DiClemente, C.C. (1984) *The transtheoretical approach: towards a systematic eclectic framework.* Homewood, IL: Dow Jones Irwin.

Further reading

Centre for Policy on Ageing (2008) CPA briefings: person centred approaches to care, www.cpa.org.uk/policy/briefings/person_centred_care_SAP.pdf , accessed 9 December 2014.

Sanderson, H. (2000) Person centred care planning: key features and approaches, www.familiesleadingplanning.co.uk/Documents/PCP%20Key%20Features%20and%20Styles.pdf, accessed 9 December 2014.

6 Partnership working

Introduction

This chapter is about partnership working, and it may be assumed that this is something that we already carry out as a matter of routine. However, the cliché often applied to personal relationships also applies here – that they need to be worked at in order to be successful. Working in a manner that fosters partnership allows you to make the most of the resources, expertise, ideas and perspectives on situations that partners can offer. Furthermore, partnership working ensures that care can be effectively coordinated in an organized manner and helps to ensure that changes are rapidly identified and acted upon.

In this chapter we will consider the role of partnership working in assessment and the important contribution that this makes in translating service users' needs into care plans and interventions that effectively meet identified needs.

By the end of this chapter the reader will have:

- considered a definition of partnership working in mental health nursing
- gained an insight into partnership working with service users
- reflected on working with carers as partners in service users' care
- reflected on how we approach partnership working with other healthcare professionals.

A definition and understanding of partnership working

Effective partnership ensures that the service user feels their needs are understood, their concerns are listened to, and that services are accessible. It also helps create a well-organized, effectively coordinated and seamless care plan that ensures the service user receives consistent input, communication and feedback on their care, and that the care plan is regularly and comprehensively reviewed. Often where complaints occur, or there is dissatisfaction with services, it is not because an adequate service for the need does not exist, or that there is a lack of resources (although this is sometimes the case) but because different parts of the service are not working together or talking to each other.

Partnership working involves effective liaison, engagement and communication with others, and managing different types of relationships with a range of people. Too often this complex skill is either taken for granted, underestimated or not prioritized to the detriment of service users' care.

Q: Which of the scenarios below is not an example of partnership working?

- *Involving, referring to or finding out about a new service that your organization does not generally work with.*
- *Being patient with bureaucracy to get the services that your service user needs.*
- *Making calls to different people to get to the person that you want.*
- *Persevering, listening to, empathizing with and patiently hearing the concerns of the service user or partner or carer who cannot seem to decide what they want.*
- *Finding the courage to present a different view to someone who you may see as more skilled, more knowledgeable or more powerful than you, and advocating on behalf of your service user.*
- *Trying to understand the different approach of another professional, and explaining your perspective in a way that allows you to effectively liaise with that professional.*

A: *All of the above are examples of partnership working. They all involve the mental health nurse working flexibly yet also with initiative, integrity, courage and an awareness of their responsibility and accountability (Cummings and Bennett, 2012). While these are good examples of practice that deserve praise, they may often go unnoticed or not be credited. Despite this, the most important thing is that they are recognized by service users.*

Partnership working with service users

Working effectively with service users involves good communication, meaningful collaboration and a genuine commitment on the part of the mental health nurse to building a functioning rapport (see Chapter 3, pp. 28–30). This is not always the same as 'getting on with each other'. In our personal lives we may instinctively form a rapport spontaneously with another person which requires little effort on our part, other than to 'be ourselves'. Yet even then often the most valuable and powerful relationships are those with people that have widely differing viewpoints to us, as they offer different and fresh perspectives. These relationships can take effort to maintain yet we are rewarded for our perseverance. Frequently this is the case in mental health settings, where the person may be reluctant to engage with mental health services, have beliefs that contrast with those held by just about everyone else (see Chapter 12, pp. 114–8), or be detained under a section of the Mental Health Act (1983, reviewed 2007).

Establishing a partnership with a person in mental health settings can be challenging and requires effective interpersonal skills, commitment and self-awareness, as well as integrity and a sense of purpose and values. These relationships are comprised of a complex set of attributes where the mental health nurse needs at times to be challenging but also demonstrate empathy and identification, support and trust while believing in the person and being committed to taking them forward in their recovery. Establishing this balance can be difficult, as on the one hand it involves genuine engagement and emotional investment, yet at the same time it requires the objectivity to be able to assess the situation and know how to help in a meaningful manner.

When establishing partnerships the following tips may be helpful.

Often people surprise us by their capabilities. Think of a time when someone achieved something you thought they never would. How do you feel now about having doubted them? What difference will that make to you in working with service users?

Ask your mentor, or a person that you trust and who knows you well to say which of the following qualities most applies to you and also which you need to work on:

- empathy
- support
- trust.

Now think of some actions you might carry out to develop in this area. For example, if I need to work on empathy I might consciously try and visualize being and living the life of the person and then later on reflect on whether I feel a stronger sense of identity with them. If I am working on support, I would be consciously reflecting on how often I demonstrate support to service users in assessments. Or asking for feedback from my mentor. While if working on trust, I might pay closer attention to how trusting I feel about others, and when this is greater or less, and any factors that characterize these situations.

Now mark in your calendar or diary a date some time in the future that gives you long enough to establish your new learning and reflect on whether you have made progress. If you have not then reconsider how you will address the learning need. However, if you have succeeded then look at another of the characteristics listed above and see if you can make further progress.

Q: From your experience, consider when you have felt that a professional has formed a good partnership with you that you have found helpful to you and memorable. This can be from a healthcare setting, or from school, work, or another area of your life. The examples below illustrate the impact that good partnerships can have.

A:

Example 1: *a call handler from the ambulance service stayed on the line with me and talked to me for 20 minutes while I waited for the ambulance to arrive for my relative who was very unwell and had overdosed. I felt they understood my fear and anxiety in this situation.*

Example 2: *I experienced exam nerves, and a teacher I happened to mention this to while waiting to go into the exam said they experienced exam nerves as well when they were young and also that they hadn't slept the night before or been able to eat breakfast. It made me feel better and reduced my nerves just knowing that they understood and someone else had been in my place.*

A further consideration in effective partnership working is differences in power. Power is not a tangible attribute that can be seen, but exists in the relationships between people. Historically, power imbalances between mental health professionals and service users have been noted to have a particularly detrimental influence on therapeutic relationships due to a lack of collaboration and little emphasis on partnership working (Goffman, 1961; Foucault, 2005). In addition, in contemporary settings mental health nurses, unlike other healthcare professionals, sometimes have to carry out actions that may not be in accordance with the service user's wishes at that time. This can happen, for example, in order to provide care that is in accordance with a person's best interests where the person is detained under the Mental Health Act (1983, reviewed 2007). This is only carried out in accordance with the requirements of the law, and instigated to protect the service user's safety, mental health and well-being, and that of the wider public. There is also an emphasis on using the least restrictive legal sanction, and on making every effort to inform service users of their statutory rights, and working in a manner that at all times promotes the service user's mental health and well-being consistent with the NMC code (NMC, 2015).

In fact, just as frequently, as a result of the effective interpersonal and engagement skills of mental health nurses, the possibility of a person being detained under the Mental Health Act is avoided. Therefore, central to effective and inclusive partnership working with service users is wherever possible that mental health nurses seek to reduce inequalities in power but also, where these do exist, perhaps out of necessity as a result of the law, work in a positive therapeutic manner with the service user. This requires the capacity for flexibility on the part of the mental health nurse, in being able to adapt the manner of their interaction with different individuals. It also requires a commitment to values-based practice that avoids the complacent use of power.

While we can never totally remove the existence or effect of imbalances in the power relationship, we can try to minimize the impact, and promote self-determination, autonomy and empowered decision making for the service user through acting in partnership with them. Often this is in the form of small acts of consideration. For example:

- making appointments when it is convenient for the service user
- asking where the service user would like the assessment to be carried out, for example at their home or on trust premises
- asking whether the person has said everything they wanted to say in the assessment meeting
- explaining the purpose of all interventions and avoiding assuming the person already knows something
- not using jargon, technical terms or 'healthcare-speak', while at the same time not patronizing the person
- working at the person's pace and not rushing
- if the person cannot decide, allowing them time to think and arranging further meetings and discussions
- regarding each service user's set of circumstances as new and unique and not assuming that interventions that have worked in the past with people in similar circumstances are the immediate answer
- providing the service user with the full range of options for their care without pressuring them to choose the option that we might prefer
- supporting the person in their chosen option, even if it is not the one we feel is best for them.

In this section of the chapter we have looked at working in partnership with the person and the necessary considerations that the mental health nurse needs to take into account in order to form effective therapeutic relationships. Next we will look at how we might develop partnerships with carers.

Partnership working with carers

Often mental health services respond defensively to the carers and significant others of service users. In some cases there are good reasons for this, for example in order to respect the service user's confidentiality. However, too often this reason is conveniently used as an excuse for avoiding sharing information with the person's family and significant others.

Carers' support and independent organizations are often regarded as mental health services' partnership provision for carers by default. These are often very proactive, committed and provide excellent services. However, the needs of some carers might not fit with the services offered by local carers' support organizations. For example, if I am a male carer in full-time employment with young children supporting a female partner with an acute mental health issue living in the community, my local carers' support organization may struggle to meet my needs.

However, it is still incumbent upon mental health services and an inherent part of the mental health nurse's role in providing comprehensive care to consider the person's family and wider social network. This inevitably involves conducting meaningful carers' assessments and developing care plans to support the carer of the person with the mental health problem. It is also necessary to be sensitive to the language used. For example, in some cases the person may be fulfilling the role of a carer yet feel that the term does not apply to them, as they are simply looking after their husband, wife or partner in the same way that they feel anyone else would.

The psychosocial intervention (PSI) approach may be useful in helping to assess the carer's understanding, experience, attitudes and beliefs, and how they experience the burden of caring for the person (Goldspink and Riordan, 2012). This can take different forms but often includes:

- Psycho-education, which comprises emotional support, knowledge and information about the condition (e.g. in the case of Frank and Anna in Chapter 15). In this way carers are supported in making sense of their situation and their experience.
- Problem-solving, addressing the burden of care and recognizing other options and ways of managing difficulties.
- Regular communication and information-sharing meetings.

Developing partnerships with carers incorporates them meaningfully in the care of the person in a manner that reduces the burden of care, yet also permits them to contribute positively to care plans.

Next we will consider working in partnership with other healthcare professionals.

Partnership working with other healthcare professionals

Commonly, mental health nursing care is carried out in all settings through working as part of a multidisciplinary team (MDT). Such teams often consist of mental health nurses, occupational therapists, psychologists, psychiatrists and social workers. In many cases MDTs operate a 'flattened hierarchy' where all views are considered and given equal priority. However, in others there are professional hierarchies based on the number of certain professionals represented within a team, or the professional seniority of an individual member of the team.

Partnership working within an MDT involves effective liaison with other members of the team, understanding their role and the value of the specialist contribution of different professionals, as well as the importance of arriving at decisions through debate, discussion and investigating therapeutic options. Effective use of MDTs ought to involve arriving at the best decision for the service user, as opposed to a situation where there is lip service consultation of the different professionals but the most powerful professionals make the final decision.

In some cases the debate between the perspectives of different professionals ensures that there is a consideration of checks and balances that reflect the contrasting specialist perspectives of these disciplines. For example, a social worker may desperately want a person to be informally admitted to an inpatient unit, as they are no longer coping in the community. In contrast, the charge nurse of the inpatient unit opposes this view as they are not clear what therapeutic gain will come from the admission. In this situation the decision is arrived at through discussion between the different professionals. However, it is important that in spite of disagreeing the different professionals nevertheless still work as partners with the person's well-being as their prime concern.

The following 'capabilities for inclusive practice' (DH, 2007) clearly illustrate the attributes that mental health nurses ought to cultivate within their practice in advocating on behalf of service users in a multidisciplinary environment:

- working in partnership
- respecting diversity
- practising ethically
- challenging inequality
- promoting recovery
- identifying people's needs and strengths
- providing service user-centred care
- making a difference
- promoting safety and positive risk-taking
- personal development and learning.

It is often said that values and principles inform the basis of the work of mental health nurses. These ought not to be seen as separate and distinct from practice. In fact, the opposite is the case and values only become meaningful when applied and tested in the innumerable complex situations that we encounter in practice. It is not unusual to be unsure what to do, or which option to take in these situations. Values perform the useful function of helping to guide the mental health nurse but also influence them in working effectively in partnership with the person, carers and significant others, as well as other professionals.

Conclusion

In this chapter we have looked at partnership working, beginning with a definition of how mental health nurses might understand and carry out this concept. Next we considered a range of different perspectives of partnership working, including working with the person, working with carers as partners and finally partnership working with other healthcare professionals.

Partnership working is often taken for granted, yet is an important role of the mental health nurse and essential if we are to deliver effective multidisciplinary care that effectively meets the needs of service users.

References

Cummings, J. and Bennett, V. (2012) Compassion in Practice. http://www.england.nhs.uk/wp-content/uploads/2012/12/compassion-in-practice.pdf, accessed 1 July 2015.

DH (Department of Health) (2007) National Social Inclusion Programme (NSIP) *Capabilities for Inclusive Practice*, www.rcn.org.uk/__data/assets/pdf_file/0008/513782/dh-2007-capabilities-for-inclusive-practice.pdf, accessed 16 December 2014.

Foucault, M. (2005) *Madness and civilization: a history of insanity in the Age of Reason.* Abingdon: Routledge Classics.

Goffman, E. (1961) *Asylums: essays on the social situations of mental patients and other inmates.* United States: Anchor Books.

Goldspink, S. and Riordan C. (2012) The carer's perspective, in N. Wrycraft (ed.) *Case studies in mental health nursing*, Chapter 20. Maidenhead: Open University Press.

NMC (Nursing & Midwifery Council) (2015) *The Code: Professional Standards of Practice for Nurses and Midwives*, www.nmc-uk.org, accessed 16 April 2015.

Further reading

National Institute of Mental Health for England (NIMHE) (2004) The ten essential shared capabilities: a framework for the whole of the mental health workforce, http://iapt.nhs.uk/silo/files/10-essential-shared-capabilities.pdf, accessed 16 December 2014.

NHS Education for Scotland (2011) The 10 Essential Shared Capabilities for Mental Health Practice: Learning Materials (Scotland), www.nes.scot.nhs.uk/education-and-training/by-theme-initiative/mental-health-and-learning-disabilities/publications-and-resources/publications-repository/the-10-essential-shared-capabilities.aspx, accessed 16 December 2014.

Royal College of Nursing (RCN) (2014) Social inclusion: inclusive practice, www.rcn.org.uk/development/practice/social_inclusion/principles, accessed 16 December 2014.

UK Government (1983, reviewed 2007) Mental Health Act, www.legislation.gov.uk/ukpga/2007/12/pdfs/ukpga_20070012_en.pdf, accessed 16 April 2015.

UK Government (2005) Mental Capacity Act, www.legislation.gov.uk/ukpga/2005/9/pdfs/ukpga_20050009_en.pdf, accessed 16 April 2015.

7 | Interventions

Introduction

Interventions are the activity phase of the nursing process of assessment, planning, intervention and evaluation (APIE) that we talked about at the beginning of Chapter 1. As the most visible part of healthcare, interventions often attract the most attention and may be seen as the focal point, yet this undermines the detailed process that goes on before interventions occur. In this chapter we will look at how interventions fit within the nursing process and the deliberation that occurs beforehand. We will then consider the range of interventions that may be used and how we might apply these.

By the end of this chapter the reader will:

- understand what an intervention is
- have considered approaches to interventions
- appreciate techniques for intervention that can be implemented with service users.

What is an intervention?

An **intervention** is a specific interaction, act of behaviour, communication or action with the intended effect of improving the service user's mental health and well-being. However, before an intervention it is important to establish the background, in terms of assessment, identifying the range of the service user's needs and planning care, agreeing what ought to be prioritized and the desired measures to be carried out. At the same time this is occurring, as discussed in Chapters 2 and 3, the mental health nurse is communicating and engaging with the service user, developing a therapeutic rapport and establishing an understanding and basis of trust – the relationship upon which interventions will be carried out.

Q: Do interventions always need to be delivered by healthcare professionals?

A: A significant role of the therapeutic relationship is to actively empower the service user to take responsibility in their lives to the greatest extent that they are able. Therefore the emphasis ought to be upon encouraging the service user to assume control, make decisions about their care and take the lead in interventions wherever possible (Barker, 2004). As a useful maxim, care ought to be 'done with' rather than 'done to' the service user. In some cases, such as the example that follows, the intervention involves collaboration and a shared activity between the service user and the healthcare professional. However, there are situations where interventions may be carried out by the healthcare professional. However, it is always necessary as part of planning interventions that there is a rationale for who carries out the activity.

While the overall aim of interventions is to improve the service user's mental health and well-being, we cannot always judge the effectiveness solely on the outcome.

Q: Can you think of a situation where this might be the case?

A: For example, a person feels anxious in busy social settings and as a result avoids being in places where there are lots of people, such as the shops. They want to begin food shopping again as a way of getting out of their home. After discussion and agreement with their community mental health nurse the service user agrees to a behavioural experiment and to be accompanied by them to a supermarket at a time when they know the supermarket is likely to be less busy. However, the supermarket was busier than expected and the queue to pay took longer than might otherwise have been expected. In reflecting on the experience, the service user felt that they had managed their fear but that it had been harder than they had expected.

The aim of the intervention here was for the service user to experience their anxiety and so the outcome may be regarded as a success. The supermarket being busier than expected and the queue taking longer than anticipated were difficulties, but these were overcome. Often, where there is doubt or anxiety, possible barriers may be viewed disproportionately. It is exactly this tendency that the experiment endeavoured to overcome. However, as with any experiment there is always the possibility that it may not produce exactly the outcome intended.

In some interventions the service user may feel worse before feeling better and it is the case that the intervention did not succeed or produce the outcome that was desired. As people differ it is also often difficult to predict the success of an intervention until it is carried out, and what works for one individual may not for another, even though their circumstances may seem to be identical. In these cases it helps to remember that being prepared to take 'positive therapeutic risk' is an important part of learning. As a result we may refer back to the process leading up to the intervention in terms of the assessment and how the care was planned, and revisit the rationales and decisions that contributed to the intervention and consider how we might use this further knowledge in the person's care in the future. Often, choosing one option that is not successful is a learning opportunity and may help us to better understand the problem by narrowing down the options to arrive at a more suitable choice.

Central to the effectiveness of an intervention is the timing, suitability and context as part of the service user's care. Therefore, interventions can be extremely brief, in the form of apparently informal conversations, words or gestures, and yet produce a powerful effect in terms of generating change and realization or the service user seeing their situation from a fresh perspective. Well planned interventions are not stand-alone acts but often form part of a more developed approach or strategy. For instance, there may be several strands of action to support the achievement of an overall goal (see the case study on Debbie, Chapter 16). In some cases an intervention may seem to occur spontaneously, as a result of the mental health nurse's 'felt response' (see Chapter 9, pp. 70–1 where we discuss 'reflection-in-action') and from a range of options a good choice is made 'in the moment'.

Approaches to interventions:

Interventions in mental health nursing include a wide range of actions that incorporate all aspects of the person's life, including their biological, psychological and sociological functioning.

Q: Under the headings of medical, physical, psychological and sociological, identify the different interventions that mental health nurses might be involved with in the care of service users in inpatient and community settings. Then look at the list below of the possible interventions and see if there are any that you have suggested that are not included or any that are mentioned that you did not identify.

A:

Medical interventions
- In inpatient settings, administering medication in accordance with the prescription. In community settings, supporting the service user to take medication and making arrangements that will help the person be able to adhere to their medication regime.
  - In both community and inpatient settings all of the actions below…
  - providing advice and information concerning the intended action(s) and purpose of the medication
  - discussing any concerns and answering questions the service user might have about their medication
  - monitoring whether the service user is taking their medication in accordance with the prescription
  - observing the service user to monitor the effectiveness of medication and evidence of side effects.

Physical interventions
- Ensuring that the service user receives physical health assessments as necessary.
- In community settings, supporting the service user to access their GP and primary care services for routine health checks and services.
- Supporting the service user to access and attend any necessary specialist referrals and appointments for treatment.
- Encouraging and where necessary supporting the service user in everyday activities of living in terms of:
  - personal hygiene, washing and dressing
  - eating and hydration
  - regular sleep pattern
  - providing health advice and information
  - supporting service users to lead an active and healthy life that will reduce the possibility of their acquiring long-term physical health issues.

(continued)

Psychological interventions
- *Forming an effective and positive therapeutic relationship with the service user.*
- *Providing psychological support.*
- *Helping the service user to recognize their strengths and positive coping resources.*
- *Supporting the service user in working towards achieving their aspirations, the goals that they value and reaching their potential.*
- *Monitoring the service user's mood and mental state.*
- *Supporting the service user in optimizing coping mechanisms and recognizing triggers that occur in relapse.*

Sociological interventions
- *Supporting service users in terms of:*
  - *housing and accommodation*
  - *financial issues and managing money*
  - *employment, training or vocational opportunities*
  - *accessing social opportunities and maintaining social networks*
  - *maintaining family networks.*

Often, health is discussed in terms of a variety of models. These range from biological, psychological and sociological to more specialized approaches such as psychosocial and biomedical. However, there are also models that emphasize a certain shared attribute of certain groups and how this can influence their experience of health – for example, in the areas of age, ethnicity, gender and socioeconomic grouping.

Q: Looking at the above, is there a model or models that you tend to identify with more than others?

While models often provide useful perspectives that act to expand and enhance our understanding of a person's situation it is important to avoid viewing health in a compartmentalized way, especially when carrying out assessments. In the next chapter we will see how relapse can be caused by a wide range of factors, including physical and psychological factors but also environmental issues. Furthermore, it is generally accepted that biological health has an effect upon mental health and vice versa and that our sociological well-being or experience of illness will also exert an impact upon our physical and mental health.

Q: Consider how you might gain an understanding of other models and approaches and develop a broader perspective on assessment.

Different aspects of health are mutually influential and viewing issues from just one perspective will lead to a limited understanding of the person's experience. If we are to understand the exact nature of the person's need then it is important not to bias our own preconceptions but to appreciate that people can experience problems in individual and different ways.

Q: Can you think of a way in which a biological problem may affect psychological well-being?

A: Among the possible answers include if I am experiencing a headache it may be evident in my behaviour and actions towards others. Whereas I may usually be talkative and friendly, in contrast I may be irritable and reluctant to talk, and this could be perceived as an uncharacteristic change in my mood. If when asked I am then unable to clearly explain the problem, perhaps due to experiencing dementia or being deeply depressed, this may cause me frustration in addition to the pain of my headache.

Often where a person has a mental health problem other health issues are attributed as directly due to that problem. In the case of the above example, if I am depressed my antidepressant medication may be increased due to a perceived further deterioration in my mood, or, if I have dementia, anxiolytic medication may be prescribed to calm my perceived agitated mood. Yet in both instances the headache is left untreated – it is not effectively assessed. The consequences of failing to accurately identify a health problem can be quite significant, and perhaps even harmful for the person's mental and physical well-being. As mental health nurses it is necessary to make every effort to communicate effectively with service users in assessing their health issues and securing effective treatment.

In the above example for headache we may substitute:

- backache
- toothache
- stomach pain
- constipation

or any number of other troubling physical ailments that all impact on other aspects of functioning.

Techniques for intervention

Interventions are identified when creating a care plan. As discussed in Chapter 5, care plans have several sections and ought to form a coherent, integrated structure. Planning care is a gradual and structured process that ought to occur over time and in collaboration and partnership with the service user. Generally, the care plan will include the following information:

- a clear identified need, or **problem statement**
- a description of the care planned **intervention**(s) or action(s)
- the **date of review** of the care plan
- the intended **outcome**, or how it will be known that each goal has been achieved
- **the date and the signature** of the service user.

A sample care plan outline is shown in Figure 7.1.

Problem statement	Intervention– actions	Date of review	Outcome(s)	Date and signature

Figure 7.1 Sample care plan

Interventions contribute to the service user's care and need to conform to several criteria. That is not to say that an intervention might not be selected on the basis that it does not fit with a specific care plan. At any one time the service user may have several concurrent care plans that have all been devised for different needs.

Example: the person has diabetes, requiring that they regularly monitor their blood sugar, take medication as prescribed and require frequent physical health checks. However they have also experienced a relapse of their long-term bipolar disorder as a result of not taking the medication for their mental health. The person may have been experiencing a low phase of their mood and have withdrawn from all social contact, leading to them losing relationships. Because they have not left their home, they have not paid their rent or utility bills for several months and are now receiving letters demanding payment that they have left unopened.

Q: Using the above example, can you identify some areas of need for which care plans could be developed?

A: Some areas of need could include:
- **Physical health** and diabetic monitoring that considers the person being able to regularly monitor their blood sugar, take their medication and attend physical health checks.
  - **Mental health** to support the person in resuming their medication for their mental health and identifying measures that will help them to continue to take it as necessary.
  - **Social contact** to support the person in regaining contact with their social support network and links in the community. Identifying protective factors and triggers that may provide early warning signs of future relapse and taking measures to prevent further deterioration (as discussed in Chapter 8 on relapse prevention).
  - **Financial issues** – the person has unpaid bills that require urgent attention and they may need support in managing this. Financial issues can also be incorporated into relapse prevention measures, if these represent early warning signs or indications of the person's deteriorating mental health.

It is helpful when agreeing an intervention with the service user to consider whether it is feasible and fits the stages of the **CARE** and **SMART** acronyms. So, for example, is the intervention:

- Centred, in terms of being agreed between the service user and the mental health nurse as a need?
- Has it been **A**ssessed as a priority emerging above other needs through collaborative discussion between the service user and the mental health nurse?
- Does the intervention that is agreed provide a **R**esponse to the need that the service user has identified and that has emerged from the assessment by the mental health nurse?
- Can the outcome of the intervention be **E**valuated?

So, in the **CARE** acronym the collaboration of the mental health nurse and the service user provides a **C**entred basis of agreement of an **A**ssessed need. The identified **R**esponse will directly address the need, the success of which is then **E**valuated.

While the person may have numerous needs, it is through negotiation and agreement between the service user and the mental health nurse that a decision is made as to which needs should be prioritized. As discussed in Chapter 5, service users may often experience challenges to the level of their motivation, due to their mental health or other factors. Yet this ought to be regarded as *part* of the process and incorporated within the assessment and planning of care.

The **SMART** acronym offers a helpful way of selecting suitable and practical care-planned measures. **SMART** stands for:

- **S**pecific – is there a clear goal?
- **M**easurable – do we know when we have reached goal?
- **A**chievable – is the goal attainable?
- **R**ealistic – is the goal reasonable within the available resources?
- **T**ime limited – can the goal be achieved within the time available?

However, it is also essential that the care-planned measure is a goal that the service user feels motivated towards and can see the benefit of achieving. They must understand how it will contribute to their recovery.

Conclusion

Interventions are an essential part of the care process, and are the result of the supporting structure of the assessment and planning of care, together with the effective implementation of communication and interpersonal skills on the part of the mental health nurse. Interventions need to be adapted and suited to the service user's specific and personal need and form part of an overall strategy or approach to care. In this chapter we have looked at how interventions may be negotiated and are mutually agreed between the service user and the mental health nurse and have discussed the CARE and SMART acronyms as useful tools for testing interventions. We shall later consider in the discussion of the examples in Section 3 of this book how different approaches to interventions can be applied.

Reference

Barker, P.J. (2004) *Assessment in psychiatric and mental health nursing*, 2nd edn. Cheltenham: Nelson Thornes.

Further reading

Callaghan, P. (2004) Exercise: a neglected intervention in mental health care? http://isites.harvard. edu/fs/docs/icb.topic253774.files/April%201%20readings/Exercise%20Callaghan.pdf, accessed 9 December 2014.

Patient.co.uk (undated) Crisis intervention, www.patient.co.uk/doctor/Crisis-Intervention, accessed 9 December 2014.

Zauszniewski, J.A., Bekhet, A. and Haberlein, S. (2012) A decade of published evidence for psychiatric and mental health nursing interventions, www.nursingworld.org/MainMenuCategories/ANAMar-ketplace/ANAPeriodicals/OJIN/TableofContents/Vol-17-2012/No3-Sept-2012/Hirsh-Institute-Arti-cle/Decade-of-Published-Evidence-for-Psychiatric-Mental-Health-Interventions.html#Haberlein, accessed 9 December 2014.

8 Relapse prevention

Introduction

The nature of mental illness means that recovery does not always follow a straight-forward path and unfortunately many people experience relapse. Often it is accompanied by apprehension, fear at the distress and upheaval that might follow, and even a sense of failure. Due to the familiarity of these feelings, relapse is unlike the first experience of a mental health problem and can be as, or even more, distressing.

In this chapter we will discuss what relapse is and how we understand it. We then consider approaches to relapse prevention, including 'wellness recovery action planning' (WRAP) and how this approach is applied in working to prevent relapses occurring and optimizing mental health and well-being.

By the end of this chapter the reader will:

- have reflected on relapse and the importance of putting preventative measures in place

- understand approaches to relapse prevention
- have gained an insight into effective techniques for relapse prevention.

What is relapse?

Evidence indicates that in a range of mental health problems, from alcohol and substance misuse to anxiety, bipolar disorder, depression and schizophrenia, there is a very high instance of relapse (MHF, 2007; Gillespie, 2010; Rodgers et al., 2012). The likelihood of future relapses also increases sharply each time the person experiences further episodes. Although relapse is never inevitable, these facts offer sufficiently compelling evidence to reinforce the view that relapse ought to be anticipated and form a central concern in assessing and planning care in mental health nursing. How mental health nurses perceive the experience of relapse and regard it in the context of the person's experience is crucial if we are to form a productive therapeutic relationship with the person. As discussed in Chapter 3, engaging effectively with the service user depends upon forming a positive rapport and developing empathy with them.

Q: Remember on page 24 in Chapter 3, you were asked who you trust and the qualities of that person that lead you to that feeling of trust. Thinking about these qualities again you may notice that they reflect an understanding and positive perception of you as a person. We all respond better to people when we feel that they understand us, believe in us, see our positive qualities and have our best interests at heart. Now think about how you might apply this same principle in working as a mental health nurse with service users.

A: There is an important difference in the boundaries in our relationships with service users, relatives and friends and it is necessary to be aware of this distinction. However, qualities such as honesty, integrity, trust and positive beliefs (such as that people can always achieve positive change and working in the person's best interests) apply in both relationship types and make a crucial positive difference when present: equally, they can undermine effective therapeutic rapport when absent. Therefore it is important to reflect on our feelings and how these are active in the therapeutic relationship.

Maintaining a sense of optimism, confidence in the person and their positive abilities and ultimately their capacity to recover is essential, even where there are ongoing problems, or recurrent episodes of distress and mental ill-health. It is important to regard relapses as setbacks or lapses, as opposed to being irreversible or placing the person beyond hope. This is something on which mental health nurses need to reflect, as we discuss in the next chapter, as their attitudes will have an influence on the service user and the therapeutic relationship.

While **relapse** is often defined as a resumption or recurrence of a mental health issue, it can sometimes be hard to identify due to the different ways in which mental illness is manifest and also because the range of factors through which it is evident.

Q: Consider how a relapse of a mental health problem might be apparent. Write down your answer, and then compare it with those identified below.

A: The factors that can lead to a relapse in mental ill-health span a range of bio-psychosocial issues which are explained in more depth below.

Among the possible indicators of relapse are an increase in the severity of the existing level of mental distress, or a return of symptoms of the mental health issue as measured against diagnostic criteria. However, in some cases the nature of the problem can change, meaning that it cannot be compared with previous episodes, or there is a transition into a new phase of the problem. Some service users with a substance use and mental health issue (commonly referred to as 'dual diagnosis') may experience one or the other problem as more significant at various times.

Environmental and social issues can also influence relapse, such as detrimental changes to the person's living circumstances – for example, the loss of accommodation or financial difficulties. The loss or absence of significant relationships can also lead to relapse – for example, through bereavement, a significant relationship ending, loneliness or social isolation and social exclusion. In some instances several factors may occur simultaneously, overwhelming the person's capacity to cope. For some people with a personality disorder, characteristic to this mental health problem are difficulties in various areas of their life, and therefore the specific nature of the issue(s) causing the problem may change; however, a common feature is that the person experiences recurrent crises or relapses due to chaotic life circumstances.

Physical and psychological health is mutually influential and experiencing a long-term physical health issue can lead to a mental health problem (Gillespie, 2010). It has also been suggested that a similar range of psychosocial disadvantages are experienced by people with long-term physical health problems and those with acute mental health problems, including (Gillespie, 2010):

- the protracted nature of the health issue
- significant impact on quality of life
- incomplete or only partial recovery
- treatment regimes that can in turn create health problems.

It is tempting to seek clear explanations for relapses. However, such an approach is contrary to the process of assessment as discussed in Chapter 1, as it risks interpreting the facts before they have been fully collated or selecting information to support a pre-conceived and biased perspective. Instead it helps to consider the factors that seem to contribute to the relapse in terms of how the service user's actions reflect their perception of the situation. In this respect we can understand more about the service user's personal understanding of their situation and this will be useful in helping them to develop effective methods of responding to the same or similar challenges in the future.

Mental illness is experienced subjectively, and for each service user the cause of their relapse is different, has a personal meaning and value, and is an individual and unique narrative. For example, the death of a pet or receiving an unexpectedly high utility bill has the potential to precipitate a relapse. In contrast, a person with a severe and enduring ongoing mental health issue may withstand the loss of their home or bereavement of a close relative and not experience any deterioration in their mental health. It may also be the case that a person who has coped in highly difficult circumstances for a prolonged period of time relapses in response to a seemingly minor event, due to the progressive depletion of their coping capacities. As discussed in Chapter 3, although we can never achieve a total understanding of another person's perspective, we will appreciate it better by empathizing and trying to understand the person's priorities and values.

Approaches to relapse prevention

Identifying features of relapse is especially useful in ensuring early access to support and preventing a problem becoming a crisis. In some cases the relapse may appear unheralded, or without any warning signs. However, relapse also often follows patterns that can be unique or specific to individuals and there may be particular precursors apparent. These could include gradual changes to the person's activities of daily living occurring over time, and will therefore be hard to detect. Such changes may be in the following areas:

- sleeping patterns (disrupted rest, or sleeplessness)
- appetite and eating (loss of appetite, overeating or an irregular eating pattern)

- daily routines (e.g. the person becoming inactive, or radically changing their activities without reason)
- social contact (social withdrawal or the loss of friends).

A range of other factors may also be significant. The list that follows identifies a broad range of aspects that might be considered in assessing the propensity for relapse:

- stopping prescribed medication and disengaging from mental health services
- pervasive low mood, or sudden mood changes and unpredictability
- increased paranoia or suspicion of others
- increased engagement in obsessive or compulsive behaviour
- agitation and irritability
- disorganized thinking and not making sense or struggling to think coherently
- greater risk-taking – for example, impetuous or dangerous acts, being reckless with money or taking sexual risks
- increased use of alcohol or substances
- greater frequency and severity of self-harm.

Environmental and social factors may also play a part. For example:

- loss of a job or redundancy
- unstable accommodation
- an accident or experience of trauma
- a combination of the above or other unfortunate events.

In some situations the service user may be unaware or unwilling to admit that they may be relapsing. Sometimes it is necessary to admit the person to an inpatient area and they may be detained under a section of the Mental Health Act (1983, reviewed 2007) for their own well-being and/or that of others.

WRAP

Relapse of mental illness by definition involves a loss of control for the person and so any way in which they can be empowered can be helpful. Perhaps the best known method for relapse prevention that focuses directly on the service user's level of control and self-determination at any one time is the 'wellness recovery action plan', also known as WRAP, which was developed by Mary Ellen Copeland (1997, 2001; Copeland and Mead, 2004). The approach was derived from her personal experience as a service user and is often facilitated as a peer-led approach by fellow service users that have experienced it and received training (Wilson and Hutson, 2013). WRAP is also often delivered in groups of service users to provide an additional form of support.

WRAP allows the service user to identify and carry out actions to support and maintain mental well-being and health through self-monitoring. The aim of WRAP is for service users to take personal responsibility for their mental health and well-being and manage their mental health through self-help, at the same time being aware of and able to access support as necessary (Copeland, 1997, 2004).

WRAP has five key principles:

- **education** – learning from experience, being knowledgeable about your mental health issue and making good decisions about your life and healthcare

- **hope** – maintaining optimism that recovery is always possible and can be sustained
- **personal responsibility** – taking action where you can with the help and support of others to manage your mental health and well-being
- **self-advocacy** – being able to gain access to the services and treatment you need and being able to live your life in the way you would wish
- **support** – being able to understand what support you need, from whom and when, and being able to support others.

(CSIP, undated; Scott and Wilson, 2011; Wilson and Hutson, 2013)

WRAP emphasizes the continuous identification of and engagement in activities that promote health and seeks to minimize the effects of those that are detrimental to mental health and well-being (CSIP, undated). When using WRAP, the service user develops a comprehensive and multi-staged set of personal plans that are adaptable to changing situations, while remaining ever vigilant of the signs and possibilities of mental ill-health. Scott and Wilson (2011) suggest that WRAP encourages the service user to plan ahead, maintain control and, by concentrating on physical and mental health, maintain mental well-being. The service user often spends 15 minutes per day reflecting on the maintenance plan and often more than two hours engaged in activities that support mental well-being. In this respect WRAP is a means of maintaining control, yet with a simultaneous awareness of the risk of losing that control (Scott and Wilson, 2011).

Techniques for relapse prevention

WRAP includes seven elements.

1 **Wellness toolbox.** A description of the person when well in both thought and behaviour (Scott and Wilson, 2011). In developing the wellness toolbox the following questions are asked:
   - What am I like when I am well and what characteristics do I feel describe me?
   - How do I feel?
   The wellness toolbox also involves measures for self-monitoring, including those that worked in the past, as well as new ones. For example:
   - talking to a friend
   - having a structure to the day
   - reflective thinking, or writing in a journal.
2 **Developing a daily maintenance plan.** In this part of WRAP the person asks:
   What do I do each day that keeps me feeling well?
   Such things include physical health-related activities and other things that also promote positive aspects of health. For example:
   - eating three healthy meals a day, and drinking water at regular intervals
   - avoiding alcohol, cigarettes and illicit substances
   - engaging in 30 minutes of moderate physical exercise.
   The plan also involves engaging in activities to reduce stress, for example:
   - taking part in a game, or a leisure activity that involves physical exercise
   - meditation or mindfulness-focused relaxation

- writing a journal or diary each day (CSIP, undated; Copeland, 1997, 2001; Copeland and Mead, 2004)

  The daily maintenance plan is supplemented by other activities that are helpful but might only be carried out every now and again as required (CSIP, undated). These include:
- going for a day out
- seeing family
- caring for pets.

Q: Looking at the above activities, list the advantages they have for promoting mental health, and compare them with the suggested answer below.

A: A possible answer might be that the group of activities that will promote physical health is also likely to enhance a sense of mental well-being. They will encourage a sense of self-regard and are likely to boost self-esteem through consciously consider-ing health. Through thinking about my health I may then foster a sense of self-regard. Other activities have an emphasis on mental health and well-being. Leisure activity and meditation are likely to reduce stress, while journal writing focuses on how the person is living their life, which is consistent with the WRAP approach.

3 **Understanding triggers.** In this stage a list is made of external and internal factors that may impact on mental well-being and lead to relapse. These differ between individuals but include:
- excessive stress, tiredness or fatigue
- interpersonal conflict, discrimination, bullying or harassment
- physical ill-health (CSIP, undated).

Measures are then identified to address the effects of the trigger in addition to the daily maintenance plan. Examples include:
- deep breathing exercises
- talking to a friend to gain support
- engaging in positive self-talk
- extra sleep (CSIP, undated: Scott and Wilson, 2011).

In a similar manner, lists of actions are generated for the two further categories below, of identifying early warning signs and recognizing when things are break-ing down. It is difficult to identify specific examples of actions for these plans, as they will be different for every person. However, at each stage these become more directive, to reflect the increasingly crisis-focused nature of the situation (Scott and Wilson, 2011).

4 **Identifying early warning signs** and a plan of action (What do I need to do less often to keep well? What changes to my mental state do I notice?).

5 **Recognizing when things are breaking down** and having an action plan (What triggers initiate a chain reaction of unhelpful thoughts, feelings or behaviours? How do I think, feel and behave?). The next plan is for when the situation has dete-riorated further.

6 **A plan to use in a crisis.** (What can I do to avoid or reduce the effect of the trigger factors and to stop things getting worse?) The crisis plan includes:
   - a description of what I am like when well
   - symptoms of becoming ill whereby I can no longer make decisions
   - a list of supporters to make decisions to ensure I get treatment, care and support
   - what I want my supporters to do for me but also actions I can carry out for myself
   - indicators for when the crisis plan is no longer needed.

7 **Post-crisis plan.** Following a crisis it is very tempting to regard the situation as resolved, and no further action being needed. However, the post-crisis period is a time of adjustment, and carrying on with life might not be straightforward. There may be physical, medical and financial consequences. These include physical problems, for example as a result of self-harm or self-neglect (see Chapter 10, pp. 91–3), medical changes as a result of feeling different on a new medication, and financial consequences through loss of earnings due to not having been able to work during the crisis. There is also the issue of returning to life even if the crisis was brief. The post-crisis plan represents a bridge between the crisis and recovery but also provides the chance to reflect on and learn from the experience. It has multiple stages, and relies on a series of questions and considerations. For example:
   - I am out of crisis and ready to use this plan when…
   - How I would like to feel when out of this crisis?
   - I would like the following people to support me…
   - What I will do to ensure that I feel safe at home is…
   - Wellness tools that I will use if I start to feel worse.

In this final section of the chapter we have considered how WRAP can provide a structured and sequenced framework to support service users in recovery and in experiencing relapse. WRAP empowers the service user at a time of vulnerability, uncertainty and fear in a manner that reflects their preferences and choices in the event of their experiencing relapse.

Conclusion

As we discussed in Chapter 4 even the most effective assessment cannot remove the possibility of risk. It is perhaps useful to regard relapse in the same manner and to understand that people living with a mental health problem are prone to exactly the same challenges of living as others in our society. Therefore the possibility of experiencing relapse can never be entirely removed, yet the WRAP approach offers the opportunity to learn and set measures in place to reduce the future effects of triggers and stressors, to recognize the service user's personal patterns and maintain their sense of responsibility wherever possible.

References

Copeland ME (1997) *Wellness recovery action plan.* West Dummerston, VT: Peach Press.

Copeland, M.E. (2001) *Wellness recovery action plan: a system for monitoring, reducing and eliminating uncomfortable or dangerous physical symptoms and emotional feelings.* New York: Haworth.

Copeland, M.E. and Mead, S. (2004) *Wellness recovery action plan and peer support: personal, group and program development.* Dummerston, VT: Peach Press.

CSIP (undated) An introduction to the WRAP: wellness recovery action planning, http://www.recoverydevon.co.uk/download/An-Introduction-to-WRAP_(CSIP).pdf, accessed 2 July 2014.

Gillespie, M. (2010) Relapse in long term conditions: learning from mental health methods, *British Journal of Nursing,* 19(19): 1236–42.

MHF (Mental Health Foundation) (2007) *The fundamental facts: the latest facts and figures on mental health.* London: Mental Health Foundation.

Rodgers, M., Asaria, M., Walker, S., McMillan, D., Lucock, M., Harden, M., Palmer, S. and Eastwood, A. (2012) The clinical effectiveness and cost-effectiveness of low-intensity psychological interventions for the secondary prevention of relapse after depression: a systematic review, *Health Technology Assessment,* 16(28), ISSN 1366-5278.

Scott, A. and Wilson, L. (2011) Valued identities and deficit identities: wellness recovery action planning and self-management in mental health, *Nursing Inquiry,* 18(1): 40–9.

Wilson, J.M. and Hutson, S.P. (2013) Participant satisfaction with wellness recovery action plan (wrap), *Issues in Mental Health Nursing,* 34: 846–54.

Reflection

9

Introduction

In all healthcare professions, reflection is encouraged so that we learn from experience and can translate this knowledge into our ongoing practice. However, in order to generate sustainable and meaningful change, reflection ought to increase what we know about ourselves, our values and principles and our skills as people as well as professionals.

In previous chapters questions have been included to encourage thought about the approach you take in different areas and the ways you can learn and improve your practice. In this chapter we will consider reflection on our experience in more depth, including the use of models of reflection, and in particular we will focus on what we learn from carrying out assessments. We will also look at how we can develop and expand our range of skills and capabilities in assessment situations in order to respond in a manner that engages effectively with the service user.

By the end of this chapter the reader will:

- have an understanding, definition and appreciation of reflection
- have considered how we reflectively learn from assessments
- be equipped to use techniques of reflection and self-awareness in assessments.

A definition of reflection

Reflection is the focused and comprehensive contemplation of a specific situation or event that captures our curiosity or attention. When reflecting we review a situation in order to better understand it and identify other interpretations, or courses of action, that might have been taken to produce different outcomes. Through reflection we are also required to question the basis of our beliefs, assumptions, values and principles.

Reflection is not just about thinking. In order to generate meaningful change and improve our practice it is necessary to implement the *outcomes* of reflection. This may be in the following areas:

- implementing changes to how we approach situations
- adopting different behaviours
- reading new information and literature
- challenging our own preconceptions
- embracing new technology and methods of learning
- seeking feedback from service users, colleagues and carers.

All of the above require a range of personal characteristics and attributes, including confidence, courage, honesty, integrity, motivation and resilience. Therefore, to be effective, reflection ought to emphasize the need for balance and not only focus on areas that need improving but also on the skills and competencies that the practitioner already possesses.

Q: What do you think are the benefits of reflection? Write down your answers and compare them to those below.

A: The benefits of reflection are:
- to learn from new experiences
- to avoid making the same mistakes
- to be sure of what works in certain situations
- to consider how we have done
- to be aware of skills and competencies
- to identify what we need to work on in order to improve our skills
- to identify alternative courses of action for solving problems
- to understand the rationales for the decisions that we make
- to better understand our own motivations and responses
- to recognize and challenge our preconceptions and assumptions
- to consider our feelings about our work and the effect that it has upon us
- to explore our values and principles and seek to move forward in our thinking
- to consolidate our overall learning and consider where we are in our professional work and lives.

'Reflection-in-action' and 'reflection-on-action'

Supporting the notion of reflection being innately linked to our practice, Shön (1983, 1987) suggests that there are two types of reflection. These are 'reflection-in-action' which occurs in the moment, and 'reflection-on-action' where we consider the event in hindsight after it has happened. Schön identifies **reflection-in-action** as responding to events in a manner that changes the outcome, even though we only later appreciate the rationale on which the action was based. Through reflection-in-action professional knowledge is developed that may be useful in practice, yet is perhaps difficult to articulate or explain.

Q: Can you think of an example of reflection-in-action in assessment?

A: Here is an example. A man's wife left him several years ago. Initially he felt very angry and became low in mood, was diagnosed with depression and, following an overdose after drinking a significant amount of alcohol and attending A&E, was admitted to an inpatient mental health unit as an informal patient. On discharge from the unit, due to his living alone, and having expressed a wish to end his life, a community mental health nurse was appointed to provide ongoing support and to continue to encourage

(continued)

him to take his medication. During the assessment meeting before leaving the inpatient unit the service user and community mental health nurse formed a positive and sponta-neous rapport, but when discussing the prospect of his life on discharge the man men-tioned that he hoped things might improve for him when his wife returned, even though she had taken steps to make the separation permanent and no longer has contact with him. The mental health nurse initially intended to ask the man how he might cope if his wife were not to return to him. However in the moment the nurse decided to tactfully say that he might need to come to terms with the fact that she would not be coming back. The man seemed to accept this thought and be less upset than might have been expected, indicating that he was perhaps aware that this was the likely outcome.

Q: Where is the reflection-in-action in this example?

A: The mental health nurse intended to respond to the man in a manner that encour-aged him to examine the possibility of his wife not returning, yet in the moment chose a more direct approach. On the one hand this involved taking a therapeutic risk, in the sense that it might have undermined the therapeutic relationship. However, when reflecting afterwards the nurse felt convinced that the quality of the therapeutic rap-port would sustain the man's disappointment at considering the reality of his wife not returning to him. In this case there is the therapeutic use of the self as a professional, combining an empathic appreciation of the service user's perspective with intuition and objective judgement.

Critics of reflection-in-action suggest that the brief time available in clinical situ-ations for us to change the course of an action or adopt an alternative approach means that we are acting on intuition, instead of reflecting. Furthermore, reflection-in-action is selective of positive evidence, because examples of reflection-in-action where the change in action leads to negative outcomes are regarded as bad judgement.

In contrast reflection-on-action occurs after the event and involves understanding the meaning of the situation, developing logical links from the facts that occurred to the underlying principles and values, before arriving at coherent outcomes and actions for practice.

Q: Can you think of an example of reflection-on-action in assessment?

A: Here is an example. In an assessment of an elderly man with dementia carried out in his home by a community mental health nurse, the man's wife took a very active role. At the time the mental health nurse was very receptive of the wife's input and grateful for the information she provided. However in writing up the assessment later, the nurse reflected that the wife often answered questions on behalf of her husband.

Q: What might be the outcomes of the wife talking on behalf of her husband?

A: The outcomes might be:
- *it may further reduce his social functioning, cognitive capacities and confidence*
- *the wife's answers to the questions might also have been different from the husband's and so the nurse might not have heard his views and been able to carry out an accurate assessment*
- *the nurse's ability to be able to assess the man's mental state, mood and cognitive functioning may have been affected.*

Q: The nurse felt guilty about not having intervened during the assessment and considered how they might change their practice in future. What actions might the nurse take, or how might the nurse change their practice, specifically with regards to this service user and more generally?

A: The possibilities in this scenario are:
- *The nurse might discreetly ensure that in future meetings they will be able to speak with the husband and ask him questions.*
- *In their general practice the nurse might consider planning assessments so that they could spend some of the time one-to-one with the service user during assessment meetings. They also need to recognize where the service user's views are not listened to, and if this is the case identify measures that will ensure that the service user's views are taken into account and acted upon.*

Critics of reflection-on-action point out that it requires time, commitment and perseverance, and many nurses are kinaesthetic learners or learn by doing rather than contemplation. In addition, **hindsight bias** can lead us to recall certain facts in situations that reinforce our assumptions or preconceptions. Often it is difficult to remember all of the salient facts that might provide an accurate and unbiased picture of events. Instead, effective reflection ought to promote a more balanced or realistic recollection of events and this might involve questioning our beliefs about situations and the meanings that we attribute to our experiences.

Approaches to reflecting on assessment

In the early stages of beginning to think reflectively it often helps to use a model to guide the process. There are many different models with a variety of features.

Q: What models of reflection have you used? What has been your experience and were they helpful in expanding your understanding of the situations on which you reflected?

In spite of the differences between models there are common aspects of reflection. For example, *the reflective process needs to achieve sufficient depth of thought to promote new learning*. Reflection is a complex, multi-layered process (Moon, 2001) that can be understood as follows:

- layer 1: the facts that were evident in one event
- layer 2: what do they mean?
- layer 3: linking the understanding that develops with other themes or concepts
- layer 4: applying the new interpretation
- layer 5: The outcomes for practice. What learning has been gained?

Example: I am on placement on an inpatient unit for adults and a female service user has been admitted due to experiencing acute anxiety. When carrying out an assessment jointly with my mentor at the beginning of the assessment I asked how she was and she responded by saying that if she was fine then she would not be on the ward. At the time I said nothing but felt very hurt, humiliated and negative towards her. After the assessment, in discussion with my mentor I considered how the service user might have been feeling at the time. Through empathically placing myself in her shoes I was able to appreciate that she might have felt that the question did not recognize her obvious feelings of distress and her comment was not directed at me personally. In future I decided that in assessments I would try and focus my questions more congruently on the situation and take account of the cues provided by the person's non-verbal and interpersonal communication as well as their verbal interaction. In addition, should a similar situation occur again I would try to take things less personally and look at situations in context. I still tend to be sensitive and need to work on this but also feel that the realization emerging from this example represented a transformation. On my next shift I saw the same person on the unit and smiled and said 'hello' and we had a brief but pleasant conversation. Her mood seemed much brighter and the encounter was a complete contrast to the previous one.

Q: Can you identify an incident in your learning where transformative outcome occurred that led to your views changing?

If you are using a reflective model, this needs to be compatible with your way of thinking. The choice of reflective model is significant as while we feel intuitively more able to connect with and to use and apply some, others may feel difficult and actually increase the difficulty of the process of reflection.

Q: Consider the reflective models that you are aware of. Which do you prefer and why? What is it about those that you prefer less that leads you to form your opinion?

Always remember that feelings need to be taken into account. Often the subject that is chosen as the focus for reflection has been specifically identified due to eliciting strong feelings or emotions. You need to feel supported, able to be open with the other people with whom you are reflecting and be able to express your emotions and feelings (Moon, 2001).

Q: Consider a situation where you felt supported in reflection and able to express how you felt about an event that was important to you.

- What made it a memorable event?
- How important was it to feel supported in enabling you to express how you felt?
- How did the other person express their support to enable you to say how you felt in terms of attitude, behaviour, acts of communication?
- What attributes will you seek to embody in your own approach in supporting other colleagues and healthcare professionals?

Reflective techniques in assessment

When carrying out an assessment it is necessary to cultivate an approach where there is a spirit of genuine curiosity that is intent upon discovery and to only form conclusions after gathering all the information. In some cases an assessment involves meeting a service user for the first time and possibly in a crisis situation. Alternatively, we may be assessing a service user who has been involved with mental health services for a long time. Both of these contrasting situations present potential challenges to our attempts to carry out an assessment free from preconceptions or biased judgements.

Q: Identify an advantage and disadvantage to both of these sets of circumstances.

A: If meeting the person for the first time in a crisis situation and with limited information due to not having preconceptions we may have a more positive and empowering approach. Alternatively their assessment may overlook something quite important that if we had known in advance we could have made sure was considered. In contrast, if we are meeting the person having read a significant amount of case history, this additional depth of knowledge about them means we can avoid having to ask quite so many questions. Yet on the other hand, previous assessments may lead us to coming to premature conclusions and decisions about care and treatment and undermine the assessment process. Therefore it is important to reflect upon and challenge preconceptions that we might have in advance of the assessment.

Where the service user has undergone multiple assessments it is necessary to view the present assessment as a new conversation and opportunity to therapeutically engage with them. Furthermore, assessment is continuous and to be effective it is necessary to challenge the assumptions we make, or facts that we unquestioningly take for granted.

Example: an adult service user has been in an inpatient area for three months after being admitted due to depression. Their mood has very slowly improved, however one day they mention to their nurse that they need new clothes, as their trousers are very loose. It emerges that over time on the unit that their nutritional intake has become less and less, so that they are hardly eating and as they were already of slight build they have become significantly underweight. The nurse discusses this with colleagues at handover and then again in the ward round and it is added to the person's care plan to monitor and encourage their nutritional intake. However the nursing staff also reflected on how, over time, they had not noticed the person's reluctance to eat or loss of weight, as this was a gradual and subtle change.

It is possible that previous assessments or observations can predispose our opinion to assume that the situation is still the same. Hence it is always helpful to consider the following questions:

- What factors have changed compared to previous assessments?
- What might it feel like to be the service user?
- How do they feel in their current environment?
- What might be their fears or concerns?

Revisiting these questions and checking with the person avoids us assuming that just because the person felt a certain way at a particular point in the past this will continue to be the case now. As time passes, circumstances change and people can feel differently.

There are a number of specific techniques that we can use to reflect on and learn from assessments. These include:

- Devise a skills inventory of your capabilities and learning needs.
- Carry out online tests to identify your personal preferred learning style and identify techniques that fit this style to increase the efficiency of your learning.
- When beginning a new placement, establish a plan with your mentor about what you need to develop in your skills in assessment. Discuss with your mentor how you can take an increasing role in conducting assessments and perhaps even identify the specific questions, or areas of questioning, where you might take the lead.
- Through agreement with your mentor, carry out assessments with other members of staff and different healthcare professionals to observe different styles of assessment.
- After an assessment, reflect upon it with your mentor or other member of staff with whom you carried out the assessment and seek feedback.
- Make time after an assessment to write down your thoughts and impressions.
- Collect appropriately anonymized examples of trust- and clinical area-specific assessment frameworks and assessment tools.
- Keep a journal and read what you write, although keep the journal safe and anonymize names and identifying details.
- Regularly update your professional portfolio with summaries or excerpts of good practice from your journal.
- While respecting confidentiality, discuss your impressions, feelings and examples from clinical practice with other students, colleagues, mentors and lecturers.
- Read and search for resources on assessment and need-specific assessment tools and their supporting evidence.

Q: Which of the above is your preferred method of reflection? Think about why this is the case and what it is about this method that you like.

Reflective exercise

Q: There are a number of methods of carrying out reflection. Can you think of two advantages and two disadvantages for each method given below? See if your advantages and disadvantages match those shown, or you may have thought of some others.

A:

Method 1: On your own in a quiet room with a laptop writing down your thoughts on an incident or situation.

Advantages
I may know my own strengths and weaknesses
I may be able to identify my limitations or learning needs

Disadvantages
I may struggle to identify new perspectives on the same situation
I may be reluctant to challenge my own conclusions

Method 2: Writing down your thoughts using a reflective model

Advantages
By following a reflective model I take the situation or event through a number of stages and arrive at a fresh understanding
Using a model will help me disentangle sometimes complicated feelings

Disadvantages
Using a reflective model requires patience and perseverance
Models rely on structure and disciplined application of each sequential state that intuitive learners may find restrictive or hard to apply

Method 3: Discussing a situation or event by reflecting with a peer

Advantages
Talking about issues helps get them in perspective
Due to being in a similar situation peers often understand the situation better than anyone else

Disadvantages
A peer may not be as challenging as another person, may tend to agree with me and my reflection may simply become an exercise in self-justification and not advance my understanding of the situation or my learning
Through not having a structure or using a framework the discussion may not be reflective in terms of identifying other interpretations

Method 4: In discussion in a peer group

Advantages

(continued)

I can access multiple perspectives and viewpoints
Sometimes the views of several people provide a sense of consensus and reassurance

Disadvantages
I would need to know the group quite well and trust them, as I may feel reluctant or vulnerable talking about an incident or situation when I may not have performed well
Sometimes groups require facilitation and organization in order to function effectively

Method 5: Reflecting with a mentor

Advantages

I may respect the mentor's views and opinions
The professional experience that the mentor possesses might be very useful

Disadvantages

Different professionals have different views and values and I may not share those of my mentor which might create conflict
In reflecting on assessment it helps to make use of as many of the above methods as possible, in order to:

- *gain multiple perspectives of situations*
- *process how we feel*
- *gain varied feedback on how we have acted*
- *understand the rationales for how different people have acted*
- *ascertain how effective the assessment was and the reasons why*
- *understand whether the assessment has been useful for the service user and if so what made it effective.*

Now reflect on an assessment and consider the viewpoints of all of the people present, for example, the service user, you as a student, your mentor. Why did they say what they did, or appear to feel how they did?

Conclusion

In this chapter we have considered the role of reflection in carrying out mental health nursing assessments. Reflecting on assessment from the outset will help to remove preconceptions and bias and ensure that we are considering the basic assumptions from which we proceed before commencing assessments. There are a range of useful and practical methods that can be used to engage in reflection effectively, including with the support of others, all to be carried out with the dual aims of developing your skills in conducting assessments and maintaining a fresh and service-user focused perspective.

References

Moon, J. (2001) PDP working paper 4: reflection in higher education learning, LTSN Generic Centre, http://reflectivepractice-cpd.wikispaces.com/Definitions, accessed 19 February 2014.
Shön, D. (1983) *The reflective practitioner.* San Francisco: Jossey-Bass.
Schön, D (1987) *Educating the Reflective Practitioner.* San Francisco: Jossey-Bass.

Common aspects of mental health issues

10 | Physical factors in mental health

In this chapter we will discuss common physical health issues. While physical health issues can have a significant impact on mental health and well-being, the exact extent varies between individuals. Through looking at aspects of physical health it is possible to see how these problems may be approached from a bio-psychosocial perspective, and how the mental health nurse might assess, plan care and identify appropriate therapeutic interventions. We commence with acute problems before looking at changes in appetite, disturbed sleep pattern, a variety of frequently occurring physical health problems, disturbed sleep pattern, self-neglect and then sexual dysfunction before considering the side effects of medication.

Acute physical health problems

Definition/context

Acute physical health problems are those that require monitoring, are ongoing and may exacerbate. They include cancer, circulatory disease, diabetes and heart problems, but also respiratory disease and strokes. In many cases the person will be on prescribed medication, have a specific treatment regime and may need regular medical or health checks.

It has been suggested that people with mental health issues have a significantly higher predisposition towards experiencing acute physical health conditions than other groups within the population. Furthermore, mortality rates from acute physical health issues are strikingly higher among people that also have a mental health issue (RCP 2010; MHF, 2011; BMA, 2014).

It is also the case that people with multiple acute physical health problems experience an increased likelihood of depression (BMA, 2014). It appears that the relationship between physical and mental ill-health is complex, multifaceted and bio-psychosocial in nature . There seems to be a mutual influence between mental and physical health, with people that are experiencing long-term acute physical health issues also being prone to mental health issues (Naylor et al., 2012; BMA, 2014).

Sociologically, the Marmot Report (2010) noted the continuation of the historical theme that there is a social gradient of health, with people living in deprived areas more frequently experiencing physical and mental ill-health than those living in more affluent environments.

It is important in assessment to view the person holistically, and bio-psychosocially. This broadens the scope of our investigation and allows for more accurate assessment, yet also prevents the person becoming stereotyped and avoids diagnostic 'overshadowing' whereby the person is seen only in terms of one primary condition (Jones et al., 2008). For example, it is sometimes the case that a person with a mental health problem who complains of physical pain may have their ailment attributed to their mental health problem, as opposed to being assessed for any physical cause.

It is also necessary to adopt a holistic perspective to the range of care interventions that the person receives. For example, it has been suggested that people with ongoing mental health problems receiving support from specialist mental health services do not receive regular physical health checks, or are not offered checks for blood pressure, cholesterol, urine or weight, or advice on healthy living and alcohol, diet, exercise and smoking cessation (MHF, 2011).

Engagement

When engaging with the person, the mental health nurse will seek to establish a therapeutic rapport. In some cases the person may focus upon their physical health but for others it may be the very last thing that they want to discuss. Therefore it is necessary to be flexible regarding the focus of discussion, and it cannot simply be assumed that because the person has an acute physical health problem they will want to talk about it, though of course they might.

Assessment

It is not necessary to be an expert in physical health conditions to provide health care to a person that has an acute physical health problem. However, before doing so it will help to talk to someone that is, or carry out background reading. This helps to understand the physical processes involved in the specific health problem and any treatments. It is also not uncommon in some acute physical illnesses, and even as a side effect of medication or treatment, for there to be commonly experienced changes to the person's mental health and an impact on the person's mental health and well-being. However, it should not automatically be assumed that certain stereotypical changes can be expected, or that the severity of the physical illness will in turn lead to acute mental health issues, as each person's experience and perspective is different.

Instead it is necessary to talk to the person and listen to their perspective, identifying what they regard as the most important issues for them, to establish how they feel about their situation. There may be a variety of different perspectives and ways of coping. For example:

- The person may be glad to know that they have a specific physical health problem which explains their symptoms and allows them to access a treatment pathway. They may be remarkably resilient. It is still possible to lead an active and fulfilling life and retain a sense of optimism, in spite of physical ill-health and even a negative prognosis.

- The person may be pessimistic about the future, lose confidence and perhaps be very cautious, leading a limited life through an exaggerated belief about the frailty of their health.
- They may be reluctant to talk about their physical health issue, find it hard to accept and seek refuge in denial, refusing to acknowledge reality.
- They may minimize the effects of acute physical illness out of bravado or selfless consideration for those whom they care for.

Care planning

We have established above under engagement and assessment that the nature or severity of the physical health problem is not necessarily influential on how the person feels about it. However it is still crucial that the process of care planning considers the extent to which the physical health problem actually does impact on the person's daily life and activities. Also, where there is a possibility of physical deterioration as a result of the problem, it is important to consider what form this might take and how the person might be able to anticipate such changes and plan ahead. The negotiation of the care plan must always involve consideration of the service user's aspirations, wishes and goals, even allowing for the confines imposed upon them by physical illness (Coad and Wrycraft, 2015).

In planning care the mental health nurse may therefore be involved, if the service user gives their permission, in liaising with carers, other healthcare agencies and professionals (e.g. adult nurses, occupational therapists, physiotherapists and unqualified carers) in discussing the person's needs, preferences and negotiating care (see Chapter 6, p. 47).

Intervention

Because of the variety of perspectives the person with the acute physical health problem may have, no specific approaches are suggested here. However, whichever options are suggested the principles underlying them ought to be the same. Promoting physical health and well-being is an essential role of the mental health nurse, while also encouraging self-confidence, and reinforcing the person's sense of autonomy, hope and resilience with regard to their mental health and well-being.

It will help to ensure that the person is informed about and understands all the aspects of their care, and is encouraged to take an active role in participating in their treatment. Their care plan may involve lifestyle and dietary changes, taking prescribed medication and perhaps receiving education if required on their intended effects and purpose. The service user may engage with therapies and access regular health checks. It will help to regularly discuss with the person the necessary healthcare interventions and medication that is suitable for them. In this way the person will understand the rationale and intended action and health benefits of these measures, and will be able to make informed and empowered decisions about their care and participate proactively in the interventions.

Relapse prevention

Continuing to communicate and liaise with other agencies involved in the person's care on an ongoing basis will promote effective multidisciplinary working, though this needs to actively and meaningfully involve the person. Regular multidisciplinary reviews of the person's mental and physical health care will also ensure that any changes are rapidly identified, and the plan of care adapted accordingly. It is also essential to devise a relapse prevention plan with the person and the members of the multidisciplinary team that identifies triggers, early warning signs of deterioration in physical health, the appropriate actions to take, who is to perform them and the signs that the deterioration has been effectively addressed.

References

BMA (British Medical Association) (2014) *Recognising the importance of physical health in mental health and intellectual disability*. London: BMA.

Coad, A. and Wrycraft, N. (in press) *CBT approaches for children and young people*. Maidenhead: Open University Press.

Jones, S., Howard, L. and Thornicroft, G. (2008) Diagnostic overshadowing – worse physical health-care for people with mental illnesses, *Acta Psychiatr Scand*, 118(3): 169–71, http://onlinelibrary.wiley.com/doi/10.1111/j.1600-0447.2008.01211.x/pdf, accessed 13 April 2015.

Marmot, M. (2010) *Fair society, healthy lives: the Marmot Review*, www.ucl.ac.uk/marmotreview, accessed 16 April 2015.

MHF (Mental Health Foundation) (2011) Physical health and mental health, www.mentalhealth.org.uk/our-work/policy/physical-health-and-mental-health, accessed 14 November 2014.

Naylor, C., Parsonage, M., McDaid, D., Knapp, M., Fossey, M. and Galea, A. (2012) *Long term conditions and mental health*. London: The King's Fund Centre for Mental Health, www.kingsfund.org.uk/publications/long-term-conditions-and-mental-health, accessed 10 April 2015.

RCP (Royal College of Psychiatrists) (2010) No health without public mental health: the case for action, RCP position statement PS4/2010, http://www.rcpsych.ac.uk/PDF/Position%20Statement%204%20website.pdf, accessed 9 April 2015.

Changes in appetite

Definition/context

We eat to maintain our body's healthy functioning. Eating regularly replenishes our stores of energy and is a necessary physiological requirement for our continued health and well-being (Lehman, 2015). Yet eating also forms a significant part of our social and cultural life. People commonly meet for meals, socialize, enjoy each other's company and have very specific dietary preferences and customs based on personal preference, culture or religious belief. Therefore eating represents a complex bio-psychosocial phenomenon.

Physically, people may experience changes in appetite due to anxiety. However, the causes can also be psychological or sociological. Psychologically, people can experience problems eating through motivation – for example when depressed. Or they may experience an eating disorder where their relationship with food indicates underlying psychological issues and the person may control their eating, eat excessively, or induce purging after binge eating by using vomiting or consuming diuretics. In other cases a person experiencing dementia may forget to eat, while a person with psychosis may also forget to eat but due to being distracted by their thoughts, or beliefs about food that lead them to not take adequate nutrition.

Sociological issues that can lead to changes in appetite include a busy or inactive lifestyle, working life, or a change in the pattern of life such as working shifts. Life events and factors such as bereavement, social isolation, financial difficulty or living in a locality where healthy food is hard to access can lead to the person no longer experiencing hunger, eating excessively or eating unhealthily.

Engagement

In order to gain a picture of the person's problem it is necessary to hear their story in their own words. Therefore listening non-judgementally will help to develop a therapeutic rapport that will inform the assessment. Being receptive to the person's viewpoint will encourage them to disclose information. Yet it is also important to treat the information that they share with respect, in order to promote confidence and trust.

For a person with dementia it may help to identify the foods they like to eat and their preferred dietary intake. It will also be useful to identify their eating pattern, as some people prefer to eat small meals frequently, while others prefer to eat at certain times of the day. If the person is unable to communicate this information it may be possible to ask a significant other or carer.

Assessment

It will help to ask the person about their regular dietary intake, over how long they have experienced changes in appetite, and any beliefs or feelings that might influence their under- or over-consumption. The person may be encouraged to keep a food diary recording their intake, however caution should be exercised where the person has an eating disorder, as monitoring their food intake may worsen the issue.

In assessment we should consider a range of bio-psychosocial issues, for example:

- age, as through life our nutritional needs change and alter
- nutritional status – for example, are they under- or overweight: this can be accurately identified by using the assessment tool below
- physical health status, mobility and ability to cater for nutritional needs
- recent life events, such as losing a partner and now living alone
- recent life changes such as retiring or losing a job
- lifestyle – for example, a person with a very physical active life requires more nutrition than a person who has a very sedentary existence
- accommodation and whether they have the facilities to provide for their nutritional needs – for example, cooking facilities, or suitable and hygienic accommodation to store and prepare food
- ability to provide for nutritional needs, through budgeting, confidence and skills in cooking
- financial issues that may prevent their being able to meet their nutritional needs.

It may help for the person to keep a diet sheet that lists their food consumption, although this may be difficult where they do not eat regular meals but snacks.

Among the standardized assessment tools are the Malnutrition Universal Screening Tool (MUST), which consists of four steps (MAG, undated):

1 Measuring the person's height and weight and body mass index (BMI).
2 Identifying the person's amount of unplanned weight loss.
3 Establishing the effect if any of acute disease.
4 From the combined results of these arriving at an overall assessment of the risk of malnutrition.

Or we may use the briefer mini-nutritional assessment (MNA) that has seven domains applied over a timeframe of the last three months and measures:

- amount of increase/decrease in food intake
- amount of weight loss
- mobility
- whether the person has experienced psychological distress
- neuropsychological problems
- BMI
- calf circumference

The person's issue may be only to do with food or one among a range of issues. Yet even where the issue is in relation to the person's eating this will not be limited to affecting just their physical state in isolation. Instead there may be sociological and psychological implications – for example, being a source of shame and embarrassment, leading to the person avoiding social situations and perhaps losing friends and experiencing a sense of low self-esteem and low mood.

In the case of a person with dementia, they may still be able to take part in the assessment. Even if this involvement is partial, or with assistance from significant others or carers, this input is empowering for the person. It is possible that, for example, the person lives alone, and is asked to keep a diet sheet, yet their memory seems unreliable, and they believe they are eating regularly and well, yet carers or family regularly find food left uneaten or discarded. In these circumstances the assessment needs to be tactfully handled, to avoid making the person feel that they have failed. When carrying out nutritional assessments in an inpatient setting with a person with dementia, it is advisable to consider the support that the person needs to avoid 'doing for' the person, as opposed to 'doing with', as providing too much support will not assess the person's capabilities or encourage independence. Furthermore, a person with dementia may also have problems with swallowing, or a motor skills deficit as a result of the condition, as opposed to an actual change in their desire for or interest in food. Finally, when carrying out the MUST or MNA it is necessary to explain to the person all of the aspects of the tool, the interventions that are being carried out and the rationale for using the tool.

Care planning

The baseline data gathered in the assessment will be considered in discussion with the person in planning their care, together with the specific circumstances of the problem they are experiencing. It may be that the person has not previously recognized they are experiencing a change of appetite, or the full extent of this issue. Using 'guided discovery' and asking the person how they understand the information emerging from the assessment will help.

In working collaboratively, the person's motivation and desire for change will be very important, together with what they perceive as the priorities and what they would like to change (Prochaska and DiClemente, 1983; Whitelaw et al., 2015). Discussing with the person how they might improve their dietary intake will help them to make choices about their care and decisions in their life as to what to change and how to achieve this transition. It will also help to consider the factors that will help change but also the possible obstacles in order to understand the person's perspective, and see the situation from their viewpoint.

In planning care for a person with dementia it is necessary to fully involve them in all decision making and consideration of the care options to provide for their needs. This may also involve the input of significant others and carers.

Intervention

Supporting the person in improving their diet may take a variety of forms, depending on the nature of the problem, yet it is also necessary that interventions are tailored to personal preferences, customs, lifestyle and financial circumstances.

Interventions may include:

- encouraging a person who does not have an eating disorder or obsession to learn about the nutritional properties of different food types, the dietary needs of people of their age, gender and developmental stage of life
- for the person who does not have an eating disorder or obsession, keeping an eating diary in order to monitor their food intake and for this to be regularly reviewed
- the person attending a healthy eating group or cookery class
- for the mental health nurse to work with the person in discussing their food shopping
- the mental health nurse helping the person look up appetizing, nutritious and inventive recipes
- the person to meet with friends to eat in a social setting
- within the realistic scope of the resources and skills available, considering how the person might try new recipes, or foods they have not previously eaten.

A person experiencing dementia's ability to function can fluctuate and vary, depending on mood, whether they are fatigued, or on other health issues. This means that at times the person may be able to eat independently while at others they may not. Also, the person's ability to communicate may vary. Therefore, in providing interventions for the person's needs it is necessary to assess constantly, so that the intervention provided effectively meets the person's level of capacity to function. Furthermore, the rate of deterioration of the person to meet their nutritional needs will also vary over time. People often value the act of eating independently, as opposed to being helped, and the loss of dignity and self-esteem that they might feel at no longer being able to carry out this task ought not to be underestimated. Therefore, it is also necessary from an ethical perspective for nursing and care staff to carefully consider the balance of providing direct care and support for the person's nutrition with continuing to empower them and maintain their independence and capacity for self-determination.

Although people's nutritional needs will vary widely, among the frequently suggested interventions include:

- Considering the environment in which the person eats. For example, a busy place with many other people may be off-putting or lead to the person becoming distracted and then not eating. It may be necessary for a member of staff to stay with the person to encourage them to eat and prevent their attention from straying.
- Providing sandwiches or finger food where the person is restless at mealtimes and wants to move around, as opposed to staying in one place.
- Providing the person with foods for which they have a specific preference.
- Providing the person with adapted beakers, cutlery and implements to make eating easier following an assessment from an occupational therapist.

- Seeking the advice of a dietician regarding foods that are high calorie and good sources of nutrition.

Relapse prevention

In agreeing interventions it will help if these promote good eating habits that are affordable, achievable without too much effort and that will fit with the person's routine and lifestyle. The easier and more convenient these measures are, the more likely it is that they will be maintained. Furthermore, as emphasized in the planning of care, if the person has identified the priority that they wish to pursue and can appreciate the value of change, then this is more likely to endure.

In the case of a person with dementia, especially if they live independently or alone, it is necessary to identify a named person who is able to tell whether the person is experiencing nutritional needs in the future, and is aware of how to access support rapidly if needed. For people with more dependent needs, who may be in inpatient or residential settings, it will help to plan for future possible deterioration in the person's ability to meet their nutritional needs.

References

Lehman, S. (2015) Nutrition – studying what we eat, http://nutrition.about.com/od/nutrition101/a/why_nutrition.htm, accessed 13 April 2015.

MAG (Malnutrition Advisory Group) (undated) Malnutrition Universal Screening Tool (MUST), www.bapen.org.uk/pdfs/must/must_full.pdf, accessed 11 November 2014.

Prochaska, J.O. and DiClemente, C.C. (1983) Stages and processes of self-change of smoking: toward an integrative model of change, *J Consult Clin Psychol*, 51(3): 390–5.

Whitelaw, S., Baldwin, S., Bunton, R. and Flynn, D. (2015) The status of evidence and outcomes in stages of change research, http://her.oxfordjournals.org/content/15/6/707.full, accessed 20 January 2015.

Further reading

Nestlé Nutritional Institute (undated) Overview, http://mna-elderly.com, accessed 11 November 2014.

Patient.co.uk: Trusted Medical Information and Support (undated) Malnutrition, www.patient.co.uk/doctor/malnutrition, accessed 11 November 2014.

Frequently occurring physical health problems

Definition/context

Frequently occurring physical health problems span a wide variety of conditions such as:

- skin problems
- recurrent coughs and colds
- headaches/migraines
- back pain
- infections
- minor viruses
- digestive disorders
- bowel problems, for example irritable bowel syndrome (IBS).

Generally these are fleeting and amenable to treatment. In most cases, though not all, while uncomfortable, inconvenient and at times painful, it is possible to continue normal functioning and everyday life with these problems. Yet where they persist, are recurrent, or there are other symptoms, further investigation is worthwhile. In the case of many major physical illnesses accessing early treatment leads to a better long-term outcome and avoids unnecessary pain and distress.

The person may also be predisposed to illness due to other issues related to physical health that are covered in other sections in this chapter such as poor appetite, lack of sleep or self-neglect. Furthermore, factors such as prolonged exposure to stress, long working hours and low job satisfaction, and social isolation are all thought to lead to the person experiencing frequently occurring physical health issues (Nakata et al., 2011). The environment can also predispose people to physical health problems – for example, living in noisy, cramped, inadequate, unsafe or damp accommodation (Marmot, 2010).

Engagement

People often experience embarrassment or self-consciousness regarding physical health problems. Therefore, adopting a discreet and sensitive approach will respect the person's feelings and dignity and encourage the development of trust and openness. In order to develop a rapport it is important to understand exactly how the problem affects the person and to ensure they feel listened to, respected and supported.

Assessment

Mental health nursing pertains to all aspects of the person's bio-psychosocial functioning and how we feel physically will impact on our thoughts, feelings and actions. Learning about the usual process of the disease by talking to a healthcare professional who specializes in physical health or reading up on the issue will help you to understand how the person is experiencing this problem. However, the causes of some physical health problems can affect people in different ways. Therefore, in seeking to understand the problem care needs to be exercised in identifying the contributing factors to avoid making mistaken assumptions. For example, tinnitus, or hearing a sound that is not caused by any physical source, yet is experienced as a realistic sensation, may cause the person to experience difficulty sleeping that will in turn impact their mood. The person may therefore initially complain of sleeplessness and low mood before the root cause of the problem is discovered.

Often the person may regard the problem as something to be tolerated and endured and may not actively seek help. For example, if living in damp accommodation the person may suffer recurrent respiratory infections or frequent colds in wintertime. In this situation it may help to support the person by considering whether they could pursue other actions that might resolve the problem or be of more benefit to their health.

Care planning

It is important to actively collaborate with the person and avoid offering prescriptive advice. Instead it is necessary to discuss the different options and identify the range of choices that are available. For example, the person may already have prescribed medication and a treatment regime. Alternatively, if they have not sought medical support it may be necessary to identify what help might be suitable. If the clinical setting is an inpatient unit it is likely that there will be readily available medical support, while in the community it may be necessary to advise the person to visit their GP.

Intervention

Advocating for the person's physical health and well-being is a significant part of the mental health nurse's role, however it is important to work collaboratively and ensure that the service user is empowered psychosocially and able to make informed choices. Therefore, providing 'psycho-education' and explaining the intended actions and positive effects of medication will demonstrate to the service user the connections between the causes of their physical health problem, and how the disease process works and the intended effect and benefits of any medication or treatment they receive. Interventions might also involve the mental health nurse attending an appointment with the service user, or helping them to discuss their accommodation with a housing association or local council.

Relapse prevention

Maintaining good physical health involves engaging in a range of activities from washing and eating regularly, to cleaning the home, but also following treatment regimes – for example, taking prescribed medication and attending health checks. Often, having a routine, or taking medication at the same time of the day – for example – can reinforce these simple self-care measures. Carrying out positive actions to preserve physical health and well-being will also have positive effects on the person's confidence, self-esteem and sense of mental well-being.

References

Marmot, M. (2010) *Fair society, healthy lives: the Marmot Review*, www.ucl.ac.uk/marmotreview, accessed 16 April 2015.
Nakata, A., Takahashi, M., Irie, M., Ray, T. and Swanson, N. (2011) Job satisfaction, common cold, and sickness absence among white-collar employees: a cross-sectional survey, *Industrial Health*, 49: 116–21.

Further reading

Dougherty, L., and Lister, S. (eds) (2010) *The Royal Marsden Hospital manual of clinical nursing procedures*, 7th edn. Oxford: Blackwell.
Nash, M. (2014) *Physical health and well-being in mental health nursing: clinical skills for practice*, 2nd edn. Maidenhead: Open University Press.
Thibodeau, G. and Patton, K. (2011) *Structure and function of the body*, 14th edn. St. Louis, MO: Elsevier.

Disturbed sleep pattern

Definition/context

Sleep is an essential human requirement, and necessary emotionally, physically and psychologically to restore energy levels, regain vitality and process events that happen to us during the time we are awake. The amount of time we sleep varies between individuals but can be anything between 4 and 12 hours per night, while it is estimated that most of us spend up to one third of our lives asleep (MHF, 2011a). Sleep is controlled by a homeostatic function called the circadian rhythm (MHF, 2011b).

The quality of sleep is more important than the length of time that a person spends in bed, and so a brief period of unbroken sleep may be more beneficial than a long period of sleep that is broken and restless. Sleep is determined by habit and routine, and poor sleep may form a pattern that can be hard to break. Difficulty falling or remaining asleep, or insomnia, can be caused by the side effects of medication, or a physical or mental health problem, but our mental state, or frame of mind, can also make our sleep pattern worse – for example, through rumination, agitation or sleeping to avoid problems (MHF, 2011b).

Engagement

Often poor sleep impacts on a person's mood and is liable to make them more irritable, changeable and impatient, and perhaps experience difficulty concentrating. In establishing a therapeutic rapport it may help to be accepting where the person has difficulty focusing on detail and be flexible and empathize and understand how the person experiences the problem. As mentioned below, if the person is unable to recall for how many hours they sleep each night, this can be recorded between sessions.

Assessment

Initially a problem with sleep may be evident in another form. For example, the person may be low in mood during the day and concerned about this, but on investigation they are experiencing poor-quality sleep. Therefore, asking about sleep ought to form part of a standard comprehensive assessment of all problems. Often people have pre-existent, or erratic, sleep problems. However, experiencing stress may detrimentally impact on sleep.

In the assessment it will help to establish the person's norms, and how many hours per night they usually sleep. As many people may struggle to recall their sleeping pattern it may be necessary for them to monitor this between sessions, and to provide feedback at a later date in the form of a sleep diary (see Appendix 1 in this chapter). It will also help to ascertain whether there are any life circumstances that have recently affected the person's sleep, for instance:

- caring for a baby or young children, or a relative
- financial issues
- living in a noisy neighbourhood
- ongoing worries
- physical ill-health and discomfort/pain
- redundancy or loss of employment
- relationship breakdown
- retirement or major life change
- unstable accommodation/overcrowding/homelessness
- working shifts or very long hours.

It may also help to consider the person's lifestyle, as they may be active later in the evening, and go to bed feeling mentally stimulated, or alternatively they may be underactive during the day, meaning that they are not tired and ready to go to sleep. Eating late in the evening may also exert an influence on sleep, as some foods contain ingredients that act as stimulants. Consuming alcohol or caffeine just before going to bed can also prevent a person from sleeping.

Care planning

Anyone who has experienced this problem will be familiar with the intense wish to rest and then frustration at not being able to sleep (MMHA, 2011a, 2011b). It is easy to feel as though nothing will help and that the measures that are commonly described as promoting sleep are obvious, have been tried and that nothing will work. The mental health nurse may be able to offer an objective perspective and help the person investigate the problem and identify measures that might help. It will help to take the person through the sleep hygiene measures suggested below to see if there are any areas of their regular pattern that need changing, or new behaviours that can be adopted that will help.

Intervention

The measures that may be used for sleep problems include:

- keeping a set routine and going to bed at the same time each night
- 'paradoxical intention', where the person experiencing difficulty sleeping stops trying and stays awake: by removing effort the person is more likely to get to sleep (MHF, 2011b).
- using the sleep diary the person completed in the assessment (see Appendix 1 in this chapter) to identify the average time that they sleep and make this their new schedule, that this then becomes a newly established pattern.

'Sleep hygiene' involves a range of measures that look at the environment within which the person sleeps and how they prepare for and respond to disrupted rest. These measures include:

- asking whether the person has a bedtime routine that ensures they gradually wind down
- the person avoiding engaging in activities that are mentally stimulating or stressful just before bed
- taking a relaxing bath or carrying out some relaxation techniques, such as relaxation exercises, consciously bringing to mind a relaxing thought, or listening to calming music
- ensuring that the bedding is comfortable and there are blackout linings to the curtains
- making the bedroom a conducive place to sleep which is comfortable and restful – it helps to remove televisions, computers and other items that might act as distractions.
- avoiding large meals, alcohol, caffeine, stimulants and nicotine before bed (MHF, 2011a) – a milky drink may help
- if sleep is disturbed in the night, again a milky drink can help, as can getting up, listening to the radio etc. rather than remaining in bed and trying to get back to sleep.

In some cases medication may be prescribed to help with sleep. Such medications are called hypnotics and include benzodiazepines (frequently diazepam is prescribed) but also in some cases temazepam and zopiclone, which is a benzodiazepine receptor agonist (MHF, 2011a, 2011b). However, these are only recommended for use for between two to four weeks and where all other treatment options have been attempted, as such drugs can lead to dependence.

Relapse prevention

Sleep is a habit which can be encouraged through developing routines and actions that are conducive with rest and relaxation. Developing and keeping good habits will help to promote a person's sleep. Where problems are encountered in the future it will help to encourage the person to reflect on their sleeping pattern and any changes they may have recently experienced, and to keep a sleep diary to assess the nature and extent of the disruption.

References

MHF (Mental Health Foundation) (2011a) Sleep matters: the impact of sleep on health and wellbeing, www.mentalhealth.org.uk/content/assets/PDF/publications/MHF-Sleep-Report-2011.pdf?view= Standard, accessed 14 November 2014.
MHF (Mental Health Foundation) (2011b) Sleep well: your pocket guide to better sleep, www. mentalhealth.org.uk/content/assets/PDF/publications/MHF-Sleep-Pocket-Guide-2011.pdf?view= Standard, accessed 14 November 2014.

Self-neglect

Definition/context

Self-neglect involves a variety of activities that include:

- personal cleanliness, self-care and hygiene
- dressing and personal appearance
- nutrition and hydration.

Often this issue is a combination of a deterioration of some or all of the above factors and is pervasive and can occur gradually and over time. The causes of self-neglect include:

- physical illness or disability
- low mood and motivation, for example in depression
- the effects of schizophrenia or psychosis
- a person experiencing obsessive compulsive disorder (OCD) and consequent hoarding
- dementia and confusion.

Engagement

Self-neglect may be apparent on meeting the person and perhaps especially if this in their home environment, as our self-care is often mirrored in the circumstances in which we live. Being discreet, considerate of the person's feelings and understanding their viewpoint is necessary, as they may be embarrassed or feel a sense of shame.

Demonstrating an interest in the person, as opposed to focusing only on their self-care will ensure that an effective rapport is developed through which it is likely that a clearer understanding of the issue will emerge.

Assessment

Standards and expectations of self-care vary widely among people and are subjective. Issues of self-care and neglect invoke dilemmas regarding capacity, the person's right to self-determination and the responsibility of healthcare professionals (Braye et al., undated). Due to the situation-specific nature of practice it is important that each case is assessed on its individual merits, and if possible as part of a multidisciplinary team discussion.

Self-neglect can occur for a number of reasons, for example social isolation, lack of motivation, preoccupation with other issues as a result of anxiety or OCD, or dementia. In order to avoid imposing our own subjective standards it is necessary to consider what factors support this impression. For example:

- Does the person appear to be unkempt?
- In what condition are their skin, hair, teeth and nails?
- Are their clothes in good condition, or stained or soiled?
- Do their clothes appear to be loose or ill-fitting, suggesting a loss of weight?
- Does the person have bodily odour?

Often the person does not accept that they are experiencing a problem. For example, a person who feels very low in mood and struggles to wash, yet is normally very proud of their appearance, may deny experiencing a problem out of embarrassment. This may be especially the case if the assessment is the first meeting, they do not know the mental health nurse well, and they may be unsure of the consequences of admitting their need, and fear losing their independence.

Care planning

It is advisable to sensitively develop a therapeutic rapport and demonstrate concern for the person, listening to them, establishing trust and confidence and promoting collaborative working. In discussing the care plan it might help to encourage the person initially to identify their desired goals and aims. It is also advisable to begin with small steps that are modest and achievable. In this way the change will be sustainable and is likely to be continued.

For a person with low mood or lacking motivation due to, for example, experiencing depression, it will help to identify a number of everyday tasks that the person carries out in their life that reflect that person's scope of activity. Then the person can rate the tasks on a graded hierarchy, ranging from those that are a chore or hard work to those that are pleasurable.

Intervention

From the list of tasks identified above the person makes a selection, combining some that are a chore with some that are enjoyable and using the positive motivation of the reward of the pleasurable activity to offset the negative appeal of the task that is hard work. (You can also make use of the activity schedule in Appendix 2 at the end of this chapter).

To begin with, to build confidence and in order to embed the activity, it helps for there to be just a few quite simple and straightforward tasks. However, as the person becomes more acquainted with this method they can add more.

Due to the range of physical and mental health issues that can lead to self-neglect, other interventions might also be chosen depending on the person's specific needs. In the case of a person whose physical capabilities are compromised it may be advisable to make a referral to an occupational therapist or physiotherapist. However, it is important to be clear on exactly what aspects of daily living the referral is requesting to be assessed, and to be aware of the role and function that these healthcare professionals perform.

Relapse prevention

Self-neglect is often the result of a long-term deterioration in the person's ability to cope. Often issues such as social isolation, lack of meaningful activity and boredom can contribute to the person losing a sense of purpose gradually over time. Therefore, while self-neglect may be addressed in the short term, in preventing relapse thought needs to be given to the contributing causes. Regular reviews of care will help to monitor progress, while developing other aspects of the care plan that promote lifestyle improvements, activity and social inclusion will help to produce sustainable improvements in self-care.

Reference

Braye, S., Orr, D. and Preston-Shoot, M. (undated) Self-neglect and adult safeguarding: findings from research, www.partnersinsalford.org/documents/self-neglect-literature-review.pdf, accessed 8 December 2014.

Further reading

Salford City Partnership (2014) Adult safeguarding guidance – self-neglect, http://www.partnersin-salford.org/asg-self-neglect.htm, accessed 8 December 2014.

Sexual dysfunction

Definition/context

While some people do not need a close relationship with a significant other, and function healthily without this aspect of their life, sexuality is an important part of healthy adult life for many people and integral to how we express ourselves and relate to those to whom we are close.

Often sexuality takes the form of a physical act in which there is an immense psychological impact in terms of how we value ourselves and others. Hence sexual dysfunction can be highly distressing and damaging to a person's self-esteem. In addition to this, the loss of or inability to achieve intimacy with a partner can lead to fractures within a relationship, to feelings of rejection and to a sense of loneliness and isolation. Clearly there is a potential impact on mental and emotional health as a result of sexual dysfunction, and mental ill-health can also contribute to physical aspects of sexual problems.

While it is not uncommon for both men and women to experience a loss of desire or appetite for sex, due to differing anatomy sexual problems manifest differently for men and women. In men, common sexual problems are erectile dysfunction or premature ejaculation (Sexuality Education Network, undated). While for women, commonly reported problems include difficulty in becoming aroused, pain during sex and difficulty reaching orgasm (NHS Choices, undated).

Engagement

Often there is a high degree of embarrassment and shame in discussing sexual behaviour. Therefore, even if the sexual issue is experienced as a very significant problem for the person, it may not emerge within the therapeutic relationship for some time. However, it is also possible that the mental health nurse may feel some embarrassment discussing sexual issues. If this is the case then it will help to reflect on the reasons why. Sexuality is a deeply personal issue, and often involves strongly held beliefs and views about what constitutes correct and responsible behaviour. Therefore, it is worth reflecting on the extent to which these beliefs influence our therapeutic work.

In engaging with the person, it is helpful to demonstrate an approach that reveals a genuine concern for them and interest in their problem, focusing on building trust and emphasizing the non-judgemental nature of the therapeutic relationship, to help the person feel able to disclose what they are experiencing. For example, not assuming, just because the service user agreed at the beginning of the conversation that they are comfortable talking about the issues, that this is always the case, and periodically checking that this remains so. Also, where the person, for example, feels a sense of guilt or shame, yet there seems to be no reason for this, it is helpful to provide reassurance that other people in the same situation may not feel this way. Where the person expresses feelings of sadness or disappointment it may help to demonstrate recognition of their feelings, with comments such as, 'I can see how this affects you.'

It is also helpful to ask only enough questions to elicit an adequate understanding of the facts of the situation. It will help to focus the discussion on the person's thoughts and feelings where possible. Listening attentively may also avoid the need for the service user to repeat information or explain things more clearly than is absolutely necessary for the mental health nurse to understand what they mean.

The service user may also prefer to use specific terms to refer to specific behaviour, as this is more objective and less personal. It may help for the mental health nurse to use the same language as the service user, providing that the sense and the meaning the person attributes to these terms is understood. Therefore it may be necessary to tactfully seek clarification as to exactly what meaning the service user attributes to certain words. The service user may also provide subtle additional expressions in terms of hints, silences and indirect comments. It is best to focus on how the person feels and be aware of subtle cues to avoid any embarrassment the person may experience regarding the physical facts of the situation.

Assessment

Assessment ought to occur within the context of a caring, confidential, safe and supportive therapeutic relationship. Due to the sensitive nature of the issue and to avoid misunderstanding, questions ought to be very clear, logically sequenced and the rationale for asking them fully explained.

Norms for sexual behaviour vary enormously between individuals, together with the meaning that people attribute to intimate acts. Therefore, while asking only what is necessary for the purposes of treatment it will help to establish what the person feels has changed, the nature of the problem and their perspective of the situation. Ascertaining the person's physical health and lifestyle profile may help to throw light on their sexual functioning. Sexuality is a multifaceted bio-psychosocial issue with overlapping aspects which exercise a mutual influence. These include:

- physical exercise/inactivity
- lifestyle
- mental health issues
- physical health issues
- prescribed medication, both for mental and physical health, and potential side effects
- use of substances and frequency of use
- weight and body mass index (BMI).

The mental health nurse needs to listen carefully and avoid coming to hasty conclusions and assumptions. If in doubt about our understanding it is necessary to tactfully double check with the service user. Risk also needs to be considered, in terms of:

- exposure to potential disease
- personal safety and that of others
- emotional and psychological harm
- possible legal issues.

Where it is felt that any of the above are pertinent the nature of the risk and any necessary further action need to be discussed with the person.

Care planning

It will help to continue to use a non-judgemental and supportive approach consistent with that used in engagement and assessment in order to build trust and confidence with the person. In common with other problems, such as disturbed sleep, the person is likely to spend a significant amount of time worrying about the issue. This in turn makes the problem worse by increasing the focus on the issue when difficulties are experienced. This may also make carrying out change difficult for the person. Therefore, it will help to patiently collaborate with the person and use guided discovery to build their sense of self-efficacy and increase their confidence, and to support them to set outcomes and positive expectations of progress.

Intervention

As a result of the assessment it may be necessary for the person to have further physical tests or treatment regarding their physical health. However, once physical health issues have been addressed, it may help to support the person in focusing on thoughts and feelings. This may take the form of removing, or blocking, negative thoughts that contribute to sexual dysfunction, and replacing these with positive thoughts. Identifying automatic negative thoughts (see Chapter 12, pp. 123–5) and supporting the person in recognizing these, challenging them and then replacing them with positive thoughts will establish more positive 'self-talk', and equip the person with tools that will improve their self-esteem and a sense of positivity. This may take some time and practice, as often negative thoughts and perceptions are ingrained and acquired over a long period of time. Through working in a focused manner on the person's thoughts it is likely that their feelings will be improved and become more positive. In addition to this, the person may be encouraged to work positively on their relationship and consider aspects that they wish to develop or improve.

Relapse prevention

The work carried out in learning the intervention techniques will support the person to internalize their own capacity to challenge negative thoughts that may contribute to sexual dysfunction. Through acquiring and learning how to use these tools in a personally meaningful way the person will gain confidence to apply them again should the same issues prove to be a problem in the future. However, it may be of use to provide the person with follow-up sessions, or the opportunity of resuming contact with the service and, due to the sensitive nature of the issue, contact with the same member of staff if possible at a later date without re-referral.

References

NHS Choices (undated) Female sexual health problems, www.nhs.uk/Livewell/Goodsex/Pages/Femalesexualdysfunction.aspx, accessed 15 November 2014.
Sexuality Education Network (undated) Erectile function: prevent and reverse erectile dysfunction, www.erectile-function.com/index.php/products-and-services/self-assessment-tools, accessed 15 November 2014.

Further reading

MIND (2013) Sexuality and mental health, www.mind.org.uk/information-support/guides-to-support-and-services/sexuality-and-mental-health/about-sexuality-and-mental-health, accessed 15 November 2014.

Side effects of medication

Definition/context

Side effects are unintended uncomfortable physical and even in some cases psychological changes as a result of taking prescribed medication, and can vary widely and become apparent in all aspects of a person's physical functioning. Although prescribed with the intention of benefiting health, even the mildest medicines are pharmacological compounds with the potential to produce side effects. Known side effects that have been reported are described in the information leaflet inside the packaging, or in the British National Formulary (BNF), yet an individual can still experience others, or new ones that have not been previously identified.

It is especially the case in mental health, where medication is given for service users' psychological health, that while being prescribed with one therapeutic purpose medication may also have an effect on an entirely different part of the body or aspect of functioning. Often the service user may not make the connection that the change is due to their medication, and therefore the mental health nurse needs to carefully observe the service user taking newly prescribed medication, or after their medication has been changed, to identify possible side effects.

Engagement

Often when people experience mental health issues their reporting of side effects may be dismissed as a feature of their illness, or a discomfort to be persevered with in order to gain the benefit of the medication. While in some cases the person can have preconceptions about their medication, or experience psychosomatic effects, it is a central part of the nurse's role to advocate on behalf of service users and ensure that they gain the best possible healthcare. Therefore, it is important to actively demonstrate concern and interest, and take the person's concerns seriously, helping them progress this issue in a collaborative manner.

Assessment

Central to accurately assessing the situation is to ask the person exactly what they are experiencing. It may be difficult for the person to articulate or explain, especially if these feelings are unusual, they have never experienced them before, and they may feel anxious or frightened. If the person is experiencing pain it is worth asking, for example, if this is intermittent or continuous, and whether in one part of their body, or a stabbing sensation, throbbing or dull ache. It may also be helpful to ask them to rate their pain on a scale of 0–10, with 0 being the lowest.

Descriptive terms may also help us understand more clearly – for example, if the person describes their vision as 'blurry', or they say they are experiencing 'pins and needles'. However, they may also use idiosyncratic terms or phrases that they understand but we need to patiently ask more about. Recognizing common precursors to the person's health deteriorating further will help us to provide care for them. For example, if the person reports that their mouth is filling with saliva and becoming watery and they suddenly feel very hot then they may be about to vomit. Alternatively, if they go very pale and say that they feel light-headed they may be about to faint, so it is advisable to get them to sit down or lie on the floor as appropriate.

It will also help to ascertain whether they have previously experienced side effects as a result of prescribed medication, or had bad experiences. The service user's view of medication is also important – for example, whether they feel that the medication is of overall benefit to them or is unnecessary.

When discussing medication with a service user, we may also gain the opportunity to observe them for other physical changes. For example:

- appearing drowsy
- agitation or restlessness
- blotchy skin or rashes
- difficulties mobilizing or balancing
- excess saliva, or dry mouth
- lack of animation in expression
- seeming hot and sweaty
- seeming unusually pale or flushed
- tremors, tics
- unusual movements, such as jerkiness or rigidity.

It will also help to identify:

- all of the prescribed medications the person is taking
- dosages

- brand names
- the particular form (e.g. tablets, caplets, liquids or other)
- the route(s) by which medications are taken
- that the medication is within date
- whether the person is taking the medication according to the prescription.

In order to obtain this detailed information it may be necessary for the person to bring their medication with them to the assessment.

According to the Glasgow Antipsychotic Side Effect Scale (GASS), it is also important to ascertain whether the person has, in the last three months:

- (men only) experienced erectile dysfunction
- (women only) noticed a change in periods
- experienced blurred vision
- experienced urinary incontinence
- experienced weight gain
- felt nauseous
- felt tender around the nipples
- experienced increased urination
- not enjoyed sex
- noticed a discharge from the nipples.

There may also be other medications that the person takes in addition to those that are prescribed. For example:

- complementary medicines
- over the counter medicine without prescription
- medicine purchased on the internet.

These can all have potent effects or react with prescribed medication, and it may not be clear what their exact ingredients are. The person may also be using illicit substances, or alcohol. If this is the case it will help to identify the amount they use and the frequency.

Other factors that will affect the person's response to medication, include:

- mental health and mood
- other known physical health issues
- age
- diet and hydration
- known allergies
- weight
- well-being in general.

Often people are prescribed multiple medications for different health problems. While side effects may be due to a combination of the above factors, it is also possible that the person may have been prescribed a drug for a long period of time and not have previously experienced any problems, yet suddenly develops side effects seemingly without cause.

Care planning

Working with the person in a supportive and facilitative manner will assist them in being able to effect change. Discussing the person's attitude regarding medication will provide an indication as to their willingness to take it, or their the reasons for being reluctant. If the person has concerns about their medication it will help to clarify these, and agree the steps to then take and the actions that should follow. Being supportive and listening, as opposed to imposing the mental health nurse's viewpoint, or attempting to argue the person around to their viewpoint is advisable. Care planning ought to be based on a collaborative commitment to joint working, and flow from a belief in empowering the person to achieve their goals. Therefore it may be necessary to discuss the current medication that the person takes for their mental health and what they might like to be different in the future and how this might be achieved.

Intervention

Among the priority measures to take is to arrange for a review of the person's medications with a medical doctor, and if the person is on multiple medication for a pharmacist to also review their regime at the earliest opportunity. The person may wish for the mental health nurse and/or an advocate and be present at the meeting to support them. It will also help to consider any other factors emerging from assessment that may influence the person's susceptibility to side effects and any necessary lifestyle changes or additional discussions that are needed.

If the cause of the side effects can be identified and the medication altered or changed then it may still be necessary to monitor the person's progress and well-being with regard to the medication they continue to use. Furthermore, it is advisable to discuss with the person their feelings about their medication. The mental health nurse also needs to discuss the intended purpose, action and therapeutic benefit of all of the person's medication, both for their physical and mental health, so they are fully informed, empowered and involved in their care. It is also important to empower the person and encourage them to self-monitor their physical health, carry out lifestyle changes and adopt measures that lead to better physical health and well-being, such as regular and healthy diet, hydration and exercise.

Relapse prevention

Throughout the engagement, assessment, planning and intervention stages of care it is necessary to be consistent and transparent with the person, to promote their mental and physical health and engender trust and confidence so that they feel able to report future experiences of side effects.

Reference

Glasgow Antipsychotic Side effect Scale (GASS) (undated) www.rcpsych.ac.uk/pdf/Taylor%20hand-out,%20GASS%20scale%20%20instructions.pdf, accessed 10 November 2014.

Further reading

Liverpool University Neuroleptic Side Effect Rating Scale (LUNSERS) (undated) www.reach4re-source.co.uk/sites/default/files/9523LJ%20r4r%20LUNSERS%20questionnaire%20v2.pdf, accessed 10 November 2014.

Appendix 1: Sleep monitoring chart

Date:

	Time went to bed	Time(s) woke up and went back to bed	Cause (if known)	Time(s) woke up	How I felt: scale of 0–10 with 0 being the lowest
Monday					
Tuesday					
Wednesday					
Thursday					
Friday					
Saturday					
Sunday					

Appendix 2: Activity schedule

Day and date:

Activity	Difficulty level (1–5)	How I felt before	How I felt doing the task	How I feel now

11 Behavioural aspects in mental health

Behaviour is the way we are in relation to others in terms of mannerisms, disposition and interaction. All behaviours represent communication, and this is inextricably linked to how we think and feel and often occurs in patterns. Behaviour often causes problems because we can form unhelpful patterns that are hard to disrupt, or produce outcomes that may create difficulties for the person in interacting effectively with other people. In this chapter we will look at different behaviours that may represent problems for a person. These include: aggressive/challenging behaviour, avoidance and lack of motivation, needing, and addictive behaviours and withdrawal.

Aggressive behaviour

Definition/context

Aggressive behaviour takes the form of comments, expressed verbal intentions, gestures and interpersonal behaviours that are outside accepted social norms and may be distressing and upsetting to others. Aggression is often a part of human interaction and communication. Frequently it is tempered, managed and mediated in relationships between people. However, it becomes a problem where it is disproportionate to the situation, is expressed in inappropriate settings and causes the person problems in social settings – for example work and close relationships. Problems may also arise in relation to the police or criminal justice system.

There are a range of causes of aggressive and challenging behaviour. These include:

- beliefs about others
- difficulties with social skills and self-expression
- learned behaviour from role models when growing up
- life experiences and influential events
- mental health issues
- personal disposition and character
- physical health issues
- school or work environment
- use of illicit drugs, substances or alcohol.

Engagement

It will help to be non-judgemental, supportive and person-centred and to make clear that the purpose of the relationship is to benefit the person and help them relate better to others. If the therapeutic relationship is non-threatening and offers benefits, then engagement is more likely, as aggressive behaviour is often a result of feeling vulnerable or challenged, and/or perceiving relationships as being unhelpful.

It is also likely that this approach may not be an instant success and it may take time for the person to develop trust. This is because the person may not be used to trusting relationships and confiding in others, and therefore it may take time for the relationship to develop. The person may also feel a low sense of worth and self-esteem and lack confidence in their ability to effect change. However, it is worth persisting with this approach even in the face of repeated rejection to demonstrate consistency and reliability, and build trust.

Assessment

Aggressive or challenging behaviour often occurs as a repeated pattern in similar situations – for example, when communicating with people in positions of authority. The person may often feel that they have not been listened to or have been misunderstood, even if this may not seem to be the case to others. In assessment it will help to ask the person to talk through a situation of their choosing where they have behaved aggressively and for them to explain their perspective. Asking how the situation appeared to them allows the person to be heard. This does not necessarily mean agreeing with the person and it may be possible to discreetly challenge their viewpoint.

The nature, extent and intensity of the aggression needs to be considered in order to understand the interaction of the person's thoughts, feelings and behaviours, together with common themes or assumptions that the person makes concerning themselves, or how they appear to others and the intentions of others towards them. It will help to adopt an active listening approach (see Chapter 3, pp. 28–9).

Care planning

Once the assessment has identified the circumstances of the person's aggressive behaviour, it is then possible to explain triggers for this behaviour. In doing so links will be made between the person's feelings and thoughts to their behaviour in a given situation. It is important to support the person, yet also encourage them to question their assumptions and actions. Carrying this out within a safe and non-judgemental therapeutic relationship avoids the aggressive behaviour becoming replicated within the relationship with the mental health nurse. The working relationship focuses on guided discovery and trust and occurs at a gradual pace in order to allow for change to occur (Stubbs and Dickens, 2008; Livestrong.com, 2013).

Intervention

Interventions will focus on supporting the person to understand the negative effects of aggressive or challenging behaviour, and to develop alternative and more productive strategies in situations that typically produce these responses. Due to low self-esteem or confidence, change can be difficult, even where the effects of existing behaviours are negative or not the outcomes the person would wish for. It will help to focus on creating the opportunity to allow the person to make change.

These may be achieved via role play, where the mental health nurse and the person act out situations where the person has behaved, or is likely to behave, in an aggressive or challenging way. Using this method the person may become aware of how their behaviour 'comes across' to others and appreciate the harmful effects of 'being on the end' of aggressive behaviour. This may lead them to consider other strategies.

Disrupting the connection between feeling frustrated and behaving aggressively and recognizing the capacity to make other choices leads to working to identify and make other behaviour choices.

Using this strategy, the person may, in an agreed situation, carry out other specific new behaviours having rehearsed these scenarios with the mental health nurse before practising them in real life. Reflecting on the outcomes of different behavioural responses offers the person a wider repertoire of behavioural choices in challenging situations and builds their confidence and self-esteem through being able to better deal with such challenging situations.

Relapse prevention

To maintain change the person may be encouraged to continue to self-monitor and recognize where they are predisposed to risk and situations that provoke the feelings that lead to aggressive or challenging behaviour. They should also come to recognize their own triggers, such as feeling stressed or overworked, being tired or unable to solve a problem. With possession of this knowledge the person can then engage other strategies, such as:

- consciously inserting pauses in encounters where the person senses that they are beginning to feel aggressive
- disengaging from the situation, even temporarily, to reduce their levels of frustration
- using positive self-talk, for example: 'I've been in this situation before and solved it without losing my temper'
- thinking calming thoughts such as 'I will soon be on holiday'
- imagining calming images, such as a warm sunny day on a beach, or taking the dog for a walk
- engaging in meditation or relaxation.

References

Livestrong.com (2013) What are the treatments for aggressive behaviour? www.livestrong.com/article/87415-treatments-aggressive-behavior, accessed 27 November 2014.
Stubbs, B. and Dickens, G. (2008) Prevention and management of aggression in mental health: an interdisciplinary discussion, *International Journal of Therapy and Rehabilitation*, 15(8): 351–6.

Further reading

Centre for Cognitive Behaviour Therapy (2011) Disorders: anger., www.cognitive-behaviour-therapy.co.za/disorders_anger.htm., accessed 27 November 2014.
Skillsyouneed (2015) Recognising aggression in others, www.skillsyouneed.com/ps/dealing-with-aggression2.html, accessed 17 April 2015.

Avoidance

Definition/context

Avoidance is associated with social inhibition through feeling inadequate and experiencing acute sensitivity to negative perceptions from others. People who experience problems with avoidance fear rejection, ridicule or embarrassment in social settings. Some theories suggest that this stems from emotional neglect, or the absence of healthy attachment to parent figures in childhood (Feel Good Time, 2012). Avoidance is regarded as a form of personality disorder (NHS Choices, 2014), and manifests itself as social anxiety. It takes the form of, for example:

- deliberately choosing work settings that involve limited contact with other people
- reluctance to be involved in close relationships
- reluctance to engage in new relationships or activities
- self-perception as socially awkward, unskilled, inept or unattractive.

The person is likely to spend significant amounts of time alone, or with a very limited range of social contacts, which can lead to poorer health in all aspects of bio-psychosocial functioning.

Engagement

Often people who engage in avoidant behaviour lack social contacts and may not regularly see others, and so the prospect of having a conversation with another person may cause them concern. It may therefore be helpful at the outset of the therapeutic relationship to clarify boundaries and mutual roles and expectations. The person may also feel that seeking help represents a failure, and be embarrassed, so it will help to frame the relationship positively, without making unfulfillable promises, and to point out the potential benefits to be gained from addressing the problem.

Assessment

In assessment it will help to focus on specific situations where the person's avoidant behaviour has been apparent. This will help the person begin to recognize the connection between their thoughts, feelings and behaviours. For example, the person may see a friend in the supermarket and experience thoughts such as 'I can't think of anything to say', or 'If I speak to them they'll think I'm boring'. This leads to feelings of anxiety, and so the person does not greet their friend in order to avoid the feared outcome.

People with avoidant behaviour can engage in self-deception as to the real motivation for certain behaviours. For instance, a person who avoids social situations is due to go out one evening after work. In spite of having time free earlier in their working day they plan meetings or work appointments that have previously overrun later on in the day, and as a result have to cancel going out. On reflection their fears about feeling awkward in social settings led to their using work engagements to make them unavailable.

In hindsight the motivation for the avoidant behaviour may be plain. However, until the active factors are pointed out the person may not realize the motivations behind their actions. In these situations it is advisable to support the person to make this discovery independently using guided discovery, helping them to recollect the situation and the factors that were active at the time.

In the assessment it will also help to ascertain the nature of the feelings the person experiences that lead to avoidant behaviour, together with the frequency, strength and extent of their fears.

Care planning

The more supportive and genuinely collaborative the working relationship, the more inclined the person will be to risk making changes. It is therefore necessary to focus on the person's positive motivation in initiating and sustaining change.

In contrast with withdrawal that is often associated with depression and a loss of motivation, in avoidant behaviour the person *misunderstands* their feelings. They do not avoid social contact with others due to an aversion to other people. Instead, a significant contributing factor in avoidant behaviour is that the person often places a high value on relationships yet feels unequal to the challenges they perceive these to represent. In reality they would like to access more social opportunities, and so may have significant motivation for change. It will help in planning care to identify the person's aspirations and hopes, as they may wish to expand their range of contacts and lead a more active social life. It is therefore important to be guided by the person in setting goals.

Intervention

Avoidance is often due to a quite palpable fear and lack of self-esteem, self-worth and self-confidence in social settings. Addressing these concerns involves the person being willing to confront their fears. In some cases it will help to build the person's confidence and perception of their competence in social settings by supporting them in carrying out behavioural experiments. For example, the person might make an appointment with a friend they have not seen for some time for a coffee, meet up and carry out the activity but record their fears and expectations before and after the event. In reflecting on the exercise the person might compare whether the event matched their feared outcomes or there was a better result.

Often 'behavioural activation' (see Chapter 14, Care plan 3, p. 148) is used whereby the person identifies situations that they avoid but also activities that they look forward to and feel confident about (Veale, 2014). An avoided activity might be meeting with several friends, some of whom the person does not know that well and feels apprehensive about. An activity that is looked forward to may be meeting with their best friend to go out for a meal. Using this method the person is able to work with their motivation and carry out activities that are perceived to be difficult, yet compensate for this by also carrying out more enjoyable activities. The person keeps a diary focused on achieving specific goals and then monitors their mood and success, or otherwise, in keeping to the schedule for their activities (Veale, 2014). It is advisable to begin with small scale changes, and to focus on actions that the person identifies as having value. In this way a hierarchy of activities is developed which will be individual and different for everyone.

Finally, it is best that medication is not used when working specifically with people who engage in avoidant behaviour, as it will address the person's symptoms, yet not the causes. Instead, working directly with the behaviour will develop the person's sense of empowerment and encourage their capacity to utilize independent coping skills.

Relapse prevention

As a long-term goal continuing to develop social interests and activities that involve contact with others will help to reduce the tendency for the person to engage in avoidant activities. Practising self-monitoring will also allow the person to notice when they begin to feel more likely to engage in avoidant behaviour, and to then use the techniques that have been learned to help them respond effectively.

References

Feel Good Time (2012) What is avoidant personality disorder (AvPD) – test, http://feelgoodtime. net/what-is-avoidant-personality-disorder-avpd-test-treatment-avoidant-personality, accessed 31 October 2014.

NHS Choices (2014) Personality disorder, www.nhs.co.uk, accessed 31 October 2014.

Veale, D. (2014) Behavioural activation for depression, http://apt.rcpsych.org/content/14/1/29. full#ref-6, accessed 1 December 2014.

Further reading

Moodjuice (undated) www.moodjuice.scot.nhs.uk/behaviouralactivation.asp, accessed 1 December 2014.

Skinner, V. and Wrycraft, N. (2014) *CBT fundamentals: theory and cases.* Maidenhead: Open University Press.

Lethargy/lack of motivation

Definition/context

Lethargy or low motivation refers to mental energy and vitality. In life it is not unusual to sometimes experience a lack of motivation. This is generally fleeting and often a response to a specific situation or task that we find uninteresting. However, for many people with, for example, depression, lethargy has a significant impact on all areas of their life and their capacity to function. Often people who are depressed or low in mood experience low motivation together with other symptoms that we discuss elsewhere in this section, for example self-neglect, negative thoughts and lack of feeling.

Lack of motivation may present as:

- having trouble getting out of bed, feeling 'unable to face the day'
- feeling overwhelmed, and not knowing where to start with tasks
- partly completing tasks, then not finishing them
- doubting own ability, feeling uncertain and a lack of confidence
- lacking the motivation to care and feeling that nothing is important
- lacking a sense of purpose, and unable to think of activities to do
- feeling a lack of energy and inner drive.

Engagement

It is important for the mental health nurse to be patient and allow the person time to think and form replies to questions. Therefore the discussion may proceed at a slower pace than usual. The person may struggle with finding the right words, and for example repeatedly use sounds such as 'mmm' and 'uhh'. They may lack animation, eye contact and expression. It can be difficult talking with a person who has trouble responding but it is important to empathize, reflect on what it must be like to be in their shoes and try to understand (see Chapter 3, pp. 25–8). It will also help to reflect on the person's achievements and positive skills and resources that they may not credit.

Assessment

In assessment it will help to get an idea of the extent of the person's lack of motivation in comparison with how they were before their current experience. In some cases it is hard to be exact, as the person's mood may have undergone a gradual decline over time. However, we can ascertain:

- how long they have been feeling this way
- what they did before but do not do now
- what they do now, in terms of the nature and frequency of activities.

It will also help to identify how the person rates their feelings of low motivation on a scale of 0–10, with 0 the lowest and 10 the highest. This provides a useful baseline against which future progress can be measured. Carrying out an assessment with a person who is lethargic can be difficult, as they may be indecisive or ask others to make choices on their behalf. This can seriously undermine the therapeutic rapport and the quality of information gathered in the assessment. Therefore it helps to adopt a focused, yet patient approach. For example, if enquiring about sleep, rather than ask the person, 'How many hours a night do you sleep?', instead ask: 'What time do you normally go to bed?' Then enquire about the time the person gets up, followed by whether these are their regular times over the last few weeks and whether their sleep is broken and if they get up in the night. In this way, through gradual, patient questioning, an accurate and detailed picture of the person's situation can emerge.

Often people who lack motivation are well aware of it and feel a sense of shame and failure. It will help to offer positive feedback regarding the person's participation in the assessment wherever possible, recognizing their contribution. For example, 'Thanks for taking part in this assessment and answering these questions.' Consistent with demonstrating empathy (see Chapter 3, pp. 25–8), it will also help to acknowledge the difficulties the person may face, for example, 'I can see that this is difficult for you.'

Care planning

In planning care it helps to build upon the rapport that has already been established in engagement and assessment. A person who is lethargic may not feel they have sufficient energy to make a commitment to activities or change due to the possibility of not succeeding. However, it helps in decision making to emphasize the person's role in making choices and decisions and to work in partnership and negotiate agreed goals. Initially the agreed care planned goals might be quite small, such as getting up by a certain time in the morning, washing and dressing, or doing the washing up. These can be viewed as 'quick wins' and ways of building the person's confidence.

Working collaboratively and involving the person equally in the discussion will identify what is important to them and what they wish to achieve. Furthermore, it will ensure that agreed activities are within the person's means and potential. It will help to quantify goals and set them in terms of what can be realistically achieved and, as above, develop a hierarchy of preferences and goals as well as identifying what the person finds challenging.

Intervention

Following the planning discussion, 'motivational interviewing' (MI) may be used. MI does not directly aim to increase a person's motivation but instead involves working with the person's feelings regarding change. It uses four principles (Miller and Rollnick, 2002; Treasure, 2004):

- expressing empathy to demonstrate understanding of the person's concern
- working with the difference between the person's values and behaviours that may not be good for the person's health
- avoiding resistance and not directly challenging the person
- promoting self-efficacy and personal confidence.

Relapse prevention

Through collaborating with the mental health nurse in developing a personalized plan the person will have undergone learning that will help to develop their motivation and may improve their confidence. The person may have also developed some functional routines that help to perpetuate motivation.

References

Miller, W.R. and Rollnick, S. (2002) *Motivational interviewing: preparing people for change, 2nd edn.* New York: Guildford Press.

Treasure, J. (2004) Motivational interviewing, http://apt.rcpsych.org/content/10/5/331.full, accessed 2 December 2014 (*BJ Psych*, 10(5): 331–7).

Further reading

Motivationalinterview.org (undated) http://motivationalinterview.o.rg/Documents/1%20A%20MI%20 Definition%20Principles%20&%20Approach%20V4%20012911.pdf, accessed 4 November 2014.

Needing/addictive behaviours

Definition/context

Addiction can be understood as the repeated and sustained use of substances, or engaging in behaviours that provide short-term gratification in spite of experiencing adverse consequences. The person commonly experiences cravings, and an intense desire in the form of compulsion. Often this is thought to apply only to substance use and gambling, however other addictions include exercise, computer games and certain foods.

Addictive behaviour is characterized by:

- lack of control over use
- preoccupation with the source of the addiction
- ongoing and sustained use
- refusal to admit there is a problem.

The causes of addiction can be explained bio-psychosocially and often these individual factors act in combination.

- Physically addictive behaviours are focused on substances or activities that produce chemicals in the brain resulting in a temporary feeling of well-being.

Furthermore, some individuals have a genomic predisposition to addictive behaviour. Often the person develops a physical dependence leading to unpleasant and sometimes acute physical symptoms if they are unable to satisfy their cravings.

- Psychologically the person strongly feels unable to cope without the substance or behaviour to which they experience addiction and often adapts their lifestyle to allow them to engage in this behaviour.
- Sociologically the person's friendship circle, lifestyle and activities may be closely linked to their addiction and this makes change difficult.

Engagement

Often people who experience addiction feel a sense of shame or embarrassment, and may have been judged or discriminated against in previous contact with health or other services and expect similar treatment again. Therefore it is important to demonstrate unconditional positive regard and an empathic approach (see Rogers' core conditions, Chapter 3, p. 26) in order to understand the person's perspective and form an effective therapeutic rapport.

While encouraging change the mental health nurse also needs to make clear that the momentum for change and decisions about the pace at which this happens ought to come from the person. This avoids the therapeutic relationship becoming a 'war of attrition' between the person and their addiction and the clinician promoting change.

Assessment

Assessment provides the opportunity to establish a baseline understanding of the extent, nature and pattern of the person's substance use or addiction. The person may provide some idea of this at the assessment meeting in terms of the nature of the addictive behaviour, and the role that it performs in their life. This can be built upon and made more focused in assessment. The person may for example keep a diary recording their addictive behaviour between sessions. Often the extent of their use or amount of time that the person spends on their addictive behaviour may surprise even them and so this tool provides a useful opportunity for the person to self-monitor their behaviour, now and moving forward.

It is also worth bearing in mind that keeping a diary may not be suitable for everyone. Many people work and lead busy lives, and it may be difficult to keep a record of their behaviour. Therefore it may be necessary to use creative methods in some cases, such as using ticks or a shorthand method of recording cravings when, for example, in a public place. Adaptability and flexibility are the key things to bear in mind here.

Care planning

The mental health nurse may encourage the person to think about their capacity for change, consider what changes they would like to make, and also how these might in turn benefit their life. However, an important factor in the care that is planned is the person's level of commitment and motivation to change. The extent to which the person wants to change may be ascertained using Prochaska and DiClemente's stages of change model (1983) (Whitelaw et al., 2015). The person's motivation may be clarified (though not increased) by the use of MI (Miller and Rollnick, 2002).

It is useful to discuss the results of the diary and negotiate targets for addictive behaviours and rules that might reduce such behaviours.

Intervention

The information from the diary in assessment can be developed by using the 4WFINDS (Skinner and Wrycraft, 2014) to identify situations When the person is predisposed to temptation, Where the person is most at risk and needs to be vigilant to avoid temptation, and What the situation is and with Whom. This will allow the person to recognize when they are at risk of temptation and disrupt the immediacy of the connection between the craving sensation and addictive behaviour.

The diary can also positively help to identify where the person makes positive progress, which increases their motivation and confidence. They may also keep a diary recording how they feel about their addiction and be able to see how this changes over time.

Among other measures that can be used with addictive behaviour are:

- the person removing themselves from the situation
- when beginning to contemplate engaging in addictive behaviour engaging in 'self-talk' and consciously reflecting upon the choices that they might make
- practising 'meditative mindfulness' to induce a sense of calmness and well-being to counter compulsions.

It may be that, for example, a person with an alcohol addiction has to visit a pub for a work-related meeting. In this case behavioural rehearsal with the mental health nurse may equip them with a range of strategies or behavioural options that they can use to avoid drinking alcohol. Technological aids such as apps that allow the person to count the units of alcohol in the drinks they consume are also effective. It may also be possible to arrange for a phone call asking the person to leave when they know they will be in a situation that exposes them to temptation.

Relapse prevention

Addiction is an ongoing issue and a challenge that people with a predisposition to become addicted face every day. Even with self-monitoring tools and the ability to identify and manage known risks, there remains the possibility of encountering unexpected situations or new challenges. It is helpful to regard further episodes as lapses rather than relapses, and to devise contingency plans for this eventuality. The specific measures that are used will vary depending on what the person feels to be suitable, the nature of the problem and the availability of local resources, but examples include:

- Having a copy of a relapse prevention and management plan listing actions to take in the event of a lapse. This might even reiterate some of the techniques that were previously learned such as mindful relaxation or positive phrases.
- A friend being willing to be contacted to discuss the situation should the person feel they are 'slipping'.
- The opportunity to access specialist services at a future date without requiring re-referral.

References

Miller, W.R. and Rollnick, S. (2002) *Motivational interviewing: preparing people for change*, 2nd edn. New York: Guildford Press.

Prochaska, J.O. and DiClemente, C.C. (1983) Stages and processes of self-change of smoking: toward an integrative model of change, *J Consult Clin Psychol*, 51(3): 390–5.

Skinner, V. and Wrycraft, N. (2014) *CBT fundamentals: theory and cases*. Maidenhead: Open University Press.

Whitelaw, S., Baldwin, S., Bunton, R. and Flynn, D. (2015) The status of evidence and outcomes in stages of change research, http://her.oxfordjournals.org/content/15/6/707.full, accessed 20 January 2015.

Further reading

Cheek, B. (2010) Motivational interviewing, http://www.gp-training.net/training/communication_skills/consultation/motivational_interviewing.htm, accessed 2 December 2014.

Clinical Training Institute (undated) Pocket guide for motivational interviewing, http://motivationalinterviewing.info/resources/CTI_MI_Pocket_guide.pdf, accessed 2 December 2014.

Hartney, E. (2014) Understanding an addict, http://addictions.about.com/od/aboutaddiction/a/Understanding-An-Addict.htm, accessed 2 December 2014.

Withdrawal

Definition/context

In contrast to avoidance, withdrawal is more passive and pertains to ceasing to pursue activities that were previously part of the person's life. For example:

- not having contact with people that the person once did
- ceasing to engage in social events and activities
- losing contact with friends and acquaintances
- not pursuing hobbies and interests
- not going out.

Withdrawal is one of the most common responses to becoming depressed, or experiencing low mood. The person who withdraws may feel a low sense of self-esteem and that they are unworthy of happiness or enjoyment, or that they are unlikeable. These beliefs may be compounded through an absence of other thoughts or stimulation and highly detrimental to how the person thinks and feels.

The person may, for example, stay in their bedroom or a safe place, withdrawal does not just refer to isolation from social contact. Alternatively it may be that the person is still frequently among others, yet ceases to interact as they once did. Often this can be subtle and hard to detect and apparent only in hindsight.

Among the frequent causes are:

- successive episodes of low or depressed mood
- experiencing a traumatic event or accident, such as a road accident
- an unfortunate life event such as bereavement or a miscarriage
- a major disappointment, or disappointments – for example, losing a job
- the gradual effect of an isolated lifestyle, perhaps due to the demands of work
- the person's stage of life – for example, partner and friends have passed away
- experiencing dementia and feeling self-aware of difficulties in communicating with others, or as a result of low mood.

Engagement

Adopting a collaborative approach from the outset, yet without becoming over-familiar, empowers the person and generates a partnership approach. In the community, a face-to-face meeting, as opposed to online, will help the person to make the choice about where to meet – for example, meeting at the person's home may feel more comfortable for them and less disempowering than going to an unfamiliar place.

Assessment

Often the nature of withdrawal is gradual and pervasive, yet when confronted with the resulting problem, the person does not necessarily appreciate the contributing causes. To identify specific instances of the problem it will help to use the 4WFINDSs approach of:

- **What** are the activities and interests that the person has withdrawn from?
- **When** did the person withdraw and in what circumstances?
- **Where** did they used to go to engage in activities and interests?
- **With whom** did they engage in these activities?

(Skinner and Wrycraft, 2014)

On this basis it may be possible to derive an understanding of how the contributing factors link together to create the problem, or develop a formulation that may help the person recognize the connections between how they think, feel and behave, and the detrimental effects of withdrawal on their mood.

Care planning

In the same practical manner, moving on from the formulation it is possible to next consider the issues that the person wants to address. Change needs to be made at a rate that is sustainable and therefore it is important to negotiate small scale steps and activities that are realistic. The person who is withdrawn may avoid making decisions, and therefore in developing the therapeutic relationship it is important to encourage them to be empowered, and to support their sense of confidence and self-determination in making decisions for themselves and about their care.

Intervention

The treatment options are varied, depending on the person's lifestyle, preferences and level of motivation (see MI, p. 108), as well as their pre-existent physical health. Examples include:

- exercise to increase physical and psychological well-being and motivation
- group therapies to provide the opportunity to meet with others that may have similar issues
- individual cognitive behavioural therapy (CBT) can help to gradually develop confidence in social situations yet with a focus on the behavioural causes of the withdrawal.

Relapse prevention

Depending on the nature of the problem, the person may require a brief period of specific input. In some cases individual booster sessions can be arranged once CBT has ended to reiterate problem-solving techniques, or sessions can be reduced in a tapered fashion. Alternatively the person may require support over a longer term.

Reference

Skinner, V. and Wrycraft, N. (2014) *CBT fundamentals: theory and cases*. Maidenhead: Open University Press.

Further reading

Feel Good Time (2012) What is avoidant personality disorder (avp) – test, http://feelgoodtime .net/what-is-avoidant-personality-disorder-avpd-test-treatment-avoidant-personality, accessed 31 October 2014.

NHS (2014) Clinical depression – treatment, www.nhs.uk/Conditions/Depression/Pages/Treatment. aspx, accessed 1 November 2014.

Veale, D. (2008) Behavioural activation for depression, advances in psychiatric treatment (APT), *Journal of Continuing Professional Development*, 14: 29–36, http://apt.rcpsych.org/content/14/ 1/29.full.pdf, accessed 11 November 2014.

12 The role of thoughts in mental health

Thoughts are also called 'cognitions', and refer to the individual's active mental processing of information. Cognitions are our perceptions of the everyday phenomena around us, and our mental activity and understanding regarding our environment and meeting our needs. Yet cognitions also include our more abstract thoughts, such as aspirations dreams, hopes, ideas, plans and wishes.

In this chapter we will discuss four aspects of how thoughts may be experienced as mental health issues: delusions and distressing beliefs, hearing voices/noises, intrusive and/or paranoid thoughts and negative thoughts. In some cases these may be stand-alone problems, and represent the only difficulty the person is experiencing. Alternatively they may be one among a range of features that all contribute to the person's experience of mental health problems.

Delusions and distressing beliefs

Definition/context

Delusions are genuine and strongly-held beliefs that the person maintains, in spite of there being overwhelming evidence to the contrary, and everyone else not agreeing with them. They can be brief in nature, or a long-term issue, and in some cases involve a very developed and complex set of ideas and meanings (Maher, 2001; Garety and Hemsley, 1997; Hartney, 2015; Purse, 2015).

Delusions occur as a result of factors such as sleep deprivation, prolonged isolation or lack of social contact and interaction with others, or as a result of illicit drug use (Hartney, 2015). However they are also often features of other mental health issues, for example psychosis, schizophrenia and bipolar disorder (Purse, 2015) and can be seen in major depression. There are a number of common features to delusional ideas centring on specific themes (see examples in Appendix 1 at the end of this chapter) and while differing widely, all share the common features of being distressing for the person and significantly impacting on their life. Some delusional beliefs are adaptations or exaggerations of a real event that has happened to the person or they have heard about. Delusions can also perform a protective role and offer an explanation of events that the person finds too traumatic to accept (Maher, 2001).

Engagement

Often delusional ideas are ingrained and hard to change. Therefore adopting a patient approach that focuses on supporting the person and developing a working therapeutic rapport is more likely to be successful. In spite of the sometimes quite unusual nature of delusions, the most surprising aspect of their experience for the person is that others do not agree with them and they feel they are repeatedly challenged about their belief. Therefore the person may feel defensive about engaging and not sure what they stand to gain from the conversation. It will help to adopt a positive approach towards them that demonstrates an interest and is non-judgemental. Directly challenging or questioning the belief should be avoided. Exceptions include where the person feels scared, unsafe or at risk due to what they believe, where it helps to provide reassurance and emphasize that your role is to support and listen to the person.

However it is still necessary to say that you, the mental health nurse, do not share the person's delusions in order to avoid collusion, or deceiving them. Therefore where the person expresses delusional beliefs or ideas, it is advisable to tactfully but briefly explain that you do not share their view. For example: 'I accept that you think that but I don't share that view.' This will establish a transparent and honest basis on which to build the therapeutic relationship.

As the rapport develops it may then be possible to facilitate an approach that encourages the person to objectively appraise the evidence concerning their beliefs (see Chapters 2 and 3 on interpersonal engagement). This empowers the person, permitting them to move forward at their own pace.

Assessment

Although it is a cliché, truth is often stranger than fiction. Therefore it is important as early as possible to establish whether there is *any* factual basis in the person's belief(s) and confirm that the delusion is incorrect by checking with other parties or agencies who have had previous contact with the person. It is also necessary to establish whether they have been prescribed medication for their mental health and if this is taken in accordance with the prescription, or, if the person has stopped, why this is the case. You should also establish whether the person has taken, or is taking, any other drugs or illicit substances.

Because of the often complex and developed nature of delusional ideas it is perhaps unrealistic to expect to form a clear understanding of their full extent quickly, or in one meeting. The mental health nurse may therefore need to temper their expectations from the assessment. In an initial meeting we may gain only a cursory insight of the person's delusions. Often a deeper understanding emerges only over time and from repeated conversations as the relationship develops, trust is formed and the person feels able to disclose this information by working gradually at their own pace.

Delusional ideas can be hard to understand as they often form a complex and elaborate system that the person takes for granted and may not think to tell someone else who does not share these beliefs. When carrying out the assessment it will help to discuss the person's beliefs and allow them to explain their view. By doing this the person is listened to and the mental health nurse better understands their ideas and how the delusional beliefs manifest themselves.

Delusions often involve words that have specific or idiosyncratic meanings with seemingly tenuous, or even no logical connection between different ideas. The person may also form conclusions that do not seem to be justified. Therefore it may be necessary to ask for clarification, or further explanation, to appreciate the way the ideas are associated. The nurse needs to achieve a delicate balance between showing curiosity about the person's belief but avoiding this inquisitiveness being interpreted by the person as them sharing these views. In achieving this balance it helps to sometimes tactfully reaffirm the understanding explained in engagement that you do not share the person's view.

In gaining an understanding of the delusion, a central theme may become apparent. In this respect, although still untrue, the delusion may have a sense of internal coherence or logic and sense.

In the assessment it may also be possible to work therapeutically with the person to explore ways in which the delusion interferes with, or limits, their life. For example, if they remain all night in their living room in a chair and avoid sleeping in case people take over their home it might be remarked how tiring this could be, or that it must be uncomfortable sitting all night in an armchair as opposed to going to bed.

When seeking to understand how the delusion impacts on the person it will help to establish the frequency and intensity, as some are fleeting or, if the ideas are ongoing, held flexibly and with only a passive interest, or experienced intensely and the person feels a need to talk incessantly about them.

Care planning

Following assessment we will have some idea of the nature of the person's delusions. In other cases though, this will only gradually become evident over time through successive conversations in which it will help to use patience and active listening skills along with interpersonal engagement (see Chapters 2 and 3). It is helpful to be open, responsive and positive, while avoiding collusion, and to demonstrate interest in and support of the person. While the thoughts that form the delusion may appear unrealistic, it is necessary to empathize and understand the emotional distress that this may cause.

In considering the planning of care it will help to adopt a future-focused approach and identify what the person hopes to achieve and what might be improved in their life. Together you can then consider how this might be achieved realistically and within the resources available.

Intervention

So far within the therapeutic relationship the emphasis has been upon building rapport, establishing a basis of trust and, while tactfully not agreeing with the person's delusions, avoiding directly challenging them. Due to the fixed nature of delusional beliefs they are often resistant to change and open attempts at doing this are likely to undermine the therapeutic relationship. Instead, at the intervention stage the mental health nurse may plan to support the person in beginning to question their delusions using guided discovery. Using this approach we may encourage the person to look at evidence supporting the belief and consider the inconvenience and discomfort it creates for them in their life.

Example: a person stays awake for as much of every night as possible in their living room with the light on out of fear that conspirators will come in and take ownership of their home. The mental health nurse might ask the person to think about whether they have ever seen any evidence of intruders and how much better they might feel being able to sleep in their bed.

It is often necessary to work flexibly with the person and avoid imposing our own expectations. Therefore in some cases it is possible that the delusions may still remain but perhaps with a reduced impact on the person. In the above case, as part of the same delusional belief the person also insisted on paying their full rent, in spite of receiving housing benefit, and had amassed a large amount of savings. Their social worker, with the agreement of the person and the multidisciplinary team, used some of this money to buy a recliner chair, so that even though the person insisted on sitting awake in their living room all night at least they were as comfortable as possible.

In cases it may be necessary to look at other measures that, while avoiding directly challenging the nature of the beliefs, may through improving the person's quality of life and well-being lead to a reduction in the influence of the delusion. For example, if the person has experienced a gradual increase in social isolation and a lack of contact with others at the same time as their delusional beliefs have increased, then measures might be undertaken to build their social involvement with others. As part of a comprehensive care plan interventions may be agreed to build the person's confidence, mental health and well-being in the long term, and establish a basis for further work. This will help to provide support for the person through the introduction of a pattern of activities such as:

- contacting friends with whom relations have lapsed
- arranging social activities
- going on courses, or learning new things such as yoga or cookery
- if suitable, meeting with family members
- renewing old hobbies or interests
- engaging in regular exercise, for example, walking or cycling.

In terms of other interventions it will help to negotiate a behavioural or thought experiment that the person is willing to participate in that would test their delusional belief. However, it must be remembered that this approach needs to be managed very carefully and with the mental health nurse offering a high level of support, as delusions feel very real to the person experiencing them, and so challenging them can be very frightening.

For the person in the above example, who is afraid to sleep in their bed because of their fear of intruders, a graded approach to the experiment might be helpful. For example, the person may be prepared to sleep in the chair in their bedroom, rather than the living room, as a first step. The next step might be to lie on the bed for a short time before returning to the chair. Although it will help if the mental health nurse supports the person, the experiment will have greater impact if the person has a central role in it and in evaluating the results. It is important that as the experiment proceeds the mental health nurse maintains a neutral stance, and does not become seen as playing a pivotal role in undermining the delusional beliefs without evidence.

It could be argued that by being willing to test the belief the person may already doubt the delusion and be willing to be swayed by the truth. Yet it is still sometimes the case that the person may continue to hold the belief in spite of being aware of the evidence by which it is disproved. Among the reasons for this are that sometimes we know that logically something is not true yet we struggle to reconcile this with how we feel. By explaining these links to the person they can be made aware of this connection, yet may still have the same belief. However the more unfeasible the belief plainly becomes, the less likely the person is to continue to maintain it and through being supported in disproving the idea over time, they may gradually feel a decrease in the strength of the belief.

Relapse prevention

Delusions are often an enduring issue and may be a persistent problem or subside to then again recur later in life. Therefore it is necessary to adopt a patient and planned approach that is focused on the longer term and considers the person's broad range of bio-psychosocial needs. By avoiding directly challenging the person's beliefs, a therapeutic rapport can be nurtured. Encouraging the person's participation in activities and exercise, engaging in new learning and education and developing their social network will provide a comprehensive range of measures. It may also be necessary that the person meets regularly with their GP or other mental health professional to ensure that help can be readily accessed in the event of their experiencing a relapse.

References

Garety, P.A. and Hemsley, D.R. (1997) *Delusions: investigations into the psychology of delusional reasoning.* Hove: Psychology Press.
Hartney, E. (2015) What is delusion? http://addictions.about.com/od/designerdrugs/g/What-Is-Delusion.htm, accessed 14 April 2015.
Maher, B.A. (2001) Delusions, in H.E. Adams and P.B. Sutker (eds) *Comprehensive handbook of psychopathology,* 3rd edn, pp. 309–39. New York: Kluwer Academic.
Purse M (2015) Delusions, http://bipolar.about.com/od/definingbipolardisorder/g/gl_delusions.htm, accessed 14 April 2015.

Further reading

Beck Institute Blog (2007) www.beckinstituteblog.org/2007/04/using-cognitive-therapy-to-treat-delusions, accessed 21 November 2014.
Kingdon, D.G and Turkington, D. (2008) *Cognitive therapy of schizophrenia,* pp. 96–119. New York: The Guilford Press.

Hearing voices/noises

Definition/context

Hearing voices can be understood as comprehending a voice or sound that has no physical source. Many of us have experienced hearing someone call our name when no one is there. However this is an isolated experience and is no comparison with what it must be like when a voice can be heard persistently or for a large amount of the time. The experience of hearing voices feels very real to the person, can be disruptive, upsetting and distressing and severely interrupts normal, daily life.

In some cases it seems that voices are speaking coherently and conducting a conversation, the voice hearer cannot predict what the voice will say next, and people can experience hearing voices in different ways (MHF, 2014). Hearing voices is a hallucination, as opposed to a delusion. The difference is that delusions (as discussed above) involve beliefs that have no factual basis, whereas hallucinations are sensations for which there seem to be no cause, and can be experienced through any of the senses (NHS Choices, undated).

There are a range of reasons for hearing voices/noises, including:

* use of alcohol, illegal drugs, and substances
* mental health issues, including bipolar disorder, schizophrenia and some forms of dementia
* physical health issues, for example dehydration, delirium illnesses and infections
* prolonged experience of stress
* insomnia.

Engagement

The experience of hearing voices can be frightening and confusing for the person. Therefore in engagement it is important to provide reassurance as to their safety, offer support and empathy, and non-judgementally listen to what they say about what they are experiencing. Demonstrating an interest in the person's overall mental and physical well-being in addition to their voice-hearing will promote engagement and establish an effective therapeutic rapport.

Assessment

As a first consideration it is necessary to ascertain whether the person receives any prescribed medication for the voices/noises and if so whether they are taking it as prescribed and if not any reasons why.

It is important to carefully consider the wording and framing of questions and comments and avoid guiding the person, asking loaded questions or imposing an interpretation of what you believe is happening, as opposed to what is actually the case. Instead, allow the person to tell you what it is that they are experiencing. It will also help to ascertain how the person feels about the voices. A thorough and comprehensive understanding will be gained by using the 4WFINDS (Skinner and Wrycraft, 2014):

- **What?** Does the voice or noise take a certain form? Is it always the same person? Are there other voices as well? Is the voice directly addressing the person? What does the voice say, or is it just a noise?
- **When?** Is the voice or noise more prominent at certain times of the day, or when the person feels a certain way?
- **Where?** Does the voice or noise occur when the person is at a certain place, or during, or following, certain situations?
- **With whom?** Does the voice or noise occur during or after encounters with certain people?

This will involve being patient, flexible and exploring the situation with the person. There may be consistent characteristics and themes to the voices/noises, however these will emerge as the discussion progresses and it is necessary to progress at a pace that suits the person.

Care planning

Planning care openly and transparently with the person allows them to feel empowered and fully included and it is helpful to be honest with them. This may include empathizing with them as to their concerns at the distressing effect of critical or negative voices/noises on their mental state. Identifying the person's goals and aspirations for care will also help in establishing positive and hopeful priorities and desired outcomes for the care plan. The mental health nurse demonstrating concern will also help in terms of shaping priorities and identifying what the person feels needs to be changed to improve their mental health.

Intervention

If the person has stopped taking medication for their voices and noises it will be necessary for a medication review to be conducted and for the mental health nurse to support and advocate for the person. The person should be advised about the intended action of the medication and any potential side effects.

Other interventions that might be used include supporting the person in recognizing the experience of hearing the voices/noises. This may apply especially if they are experiencing a voice that repeats consistent phrases, or has a particular character or persona that the person finds troubling or distressing. From this recognition and awareness the person may use distraction techniques to deflect their attention or reduce the influence of the voice. For example:

- consciously activating a pleasant thought
- engaging in an activity that is mentally absorbing
- listening to music
- practising mindfulness techniques which can help the person 'step back' from distressing thoughts.

Alternatively, if the voice is critical or mocking, for example, 'You're useless and you'll never amount to anything', the person may use cognitive restructuring and devise other more positive perspectives, such as, 'I'm a kind/caring person', or 'I'm good at . . .' that represent a contrasting, more positive perspective. However, it may take time and the use of small steps, as while the person may recognize the truth of the positive statement cognitively, it may take a while for this to feel true for the person emotionally. Therefore the mental health nurse may need to offer support and work with the person over time.

Other interventions include:

- setting a time of day, or particular period of time, to be receptive to the voice(s), to avoid experiencing them as an intrusion at other times and interfering with activities of daily living
- encouraging the person to meet with other people who also experience voices, for mutual support which is an approach championed by the service user-led movement run by the Hearing Voices Network (2014).

Relapse prevention

Often voices can be persuasive and insistent and experienced as extremely traumatic and distressing. It is helpful for the person to learn habits and techniques that they feel confident with and are able to apply in their daily life. Yet at times of stress or difficulty the person may experience relapse and the voices return. In this situation it is important to ensure that the person has a clear plan to access help. This ought to take the form of readily accessible support, whether a family member, friend or healthcare professional such as their GP or a member of the mental health team who is aware that this is their role and who can provide and/or access further help as necessary.

References

Hearing Voices Network (2014) Welcome, http://www.hearing-voices.org, accessed 25 November 2014.

MHF (Mental Health Foundation) (2014) Hearing voices, http://www.mentalhealth.org.uk/help-information/mental-health-a-z/H/hearing-voices, accessed 16 October 2014.

NHS Choices (undated) Schizophrenia – symptoms, www.nhs.uk/Conditions/Schizophrenia/Pages/Symptoms.aspx, accessed 22 October 2014.

Skinner, V. and Wrycraft, N. (2014) *CBT fundamentals: theory and cases.* Maidenhead: Open University Press.

Further reading

NHS Choices (2014) Hallucinations and hearing voices, www.nhs.uk/conditions/hallucinations/Pages/Introduction.aspx#Charles, accessed 22 October 2014.

Intrusive thoughts and paranoia

Definition/context

Intrusive thoughts are experienced as unwanted or undesirable cognitions that are often of a traumatic, violent or sexual nature. The person does not wish to experience them but feels unable to prevent them occurring and focuses upon them even though they may be distressing and unpleasant. Often as a result they may experience a high level of anxiety and, for example, insomnia, which will in turn worsen how they feel. They may also use non-prescribed drugs and/or alcohol as a means of blocking the thoughts.

Paranoia occurs where a person thinks that others intend to deliberately harm them and experiences a compelling feeling that this is inevitable (Institute of Psychiatry, Psychology and Neuroscience, 2014). Most people will experience paranoia at some time, and this is common when feeling under stress.

Engagement

The person may be irritable and unforthcoming but may also be receptive, though to a limited extent due to wishing to 'keep people at arm's length'. As a result, they may quickly become guarded and cautious over more searching issues or topics of conversation. Therefore it will help to begin to engage with the person by discussing neutral topics as a brief preface to the main conversation. This ought to be brief, as an excessively lengthy informal discussion may incite the person's paranoia by them feeling that information is being kept from them.

It is also advisable to be very clear, honest and transparent about the reason for meeting, the role of the mental health nurse in the process and the possible outcomes that may result from the meeting. If the setting is an inpatient unit and the person is obliged to remain through being legally detained under the Mental Health Act (1983, reviewed 2007), explain the nature of the section under which the person is being held, advise the person of their rights to appeal and to access to advocacy services. It is also important to emphasize that you are there to support them, ensure their safety and promote their mental health. In this way a collaborative relationship can be established that does not overlook difficulties but still seeks to form a positive therapeutic rapport.

Assessment

The irresistibility of intrusive thoughts can make the person feel powerless and unable to influence events. Therefore they may feel helpless and hopeless of ever being able to successfully challenge the thoughts. The person may also feel intense embarrassment and shame, as the content of the thoughts may be counter to their morals, personality and disposition. As a result they may feel reluctant to disclose what they are experiencing, and worry about people finding out, which may in turn increase their paranoia.

Therefore, choosing an informal method of assessment (see Chapter 1, p. 9) avoids creating the impression that information is being collected about the person that might feed into their paranoia. However, and in order to demonstrate a collaborative approach, it is still necessary to explain to the person that an assessment is being carried out. It may help to use open questions (see Chapter 1, p. 12) and a natural and conversational format may produce better results by continuing to develop and use therapeutic rapport.

The mental health nurse will assess the nature and extent of the person's intrusive thoughts. They will also consider whether the person appears not to be disclosing information or is guarded as a result of their paranoia.

In assessment it is necessary to ascertain whether the person is concordant with prescribed medication for their mental health, whether they use any illicit drugs and also the person's sleeping pattern and any ongoing stressful life events they are experiencing at that time.

Care planning

Due to the powerlessness people may feel because of intrusive thoughts and the sense of shame, embarrassment and paranoia they experience, the nature of the working relationship between the mental health nurse and the person is crucial. Adopting a non-judgemental person-centred focus that demonstrates concern for the person's well-being will continue to foster therapeutic rapport and the development of a functioning working relationship. Supporting the person to feel accepted and to understand that their experience is not unique will help to develop a sense of self-efficacy and in turn build the person's confidence and the feelings of empowerment necessary for collaborative care planning.

In planning care it will also help to adopt a patient and step-by-step approach, so that the person feels thoroughly included, which will reinforce a sense of collaborative working, openness and transparency. It will help to examine the range of options that are available and to support the person in making informed choices about their care.

Intervention

Among the interventions that might be used are (Sound-Mind.Org, 2013):

- **Revisualization:** when not experiencing the thought the person voluntarily visualizes it. In this manner the person will feel that they have some control over the thought, as opposed to passively receiving the experience. This allows the person to access other ways of appraising the thought, for example using humour, undermining it, or challenging the validity of the content to reduce the value or authority that it is perceived to hold. In addition to reducing the influence of the intrusive thought, revisualization may help to develop an alternative thought from other appraisals that the person may feel to be more representative of their viewpoint.
- **Positive self-talk:** involves reassuring notions such as that you would never carry out the content of the thought, and in spite of the thought being very strong you have the right to choose your actions.
- **Recognizing thoughts** as self-talk and no more than that, and consciously turning down the volume.
- **Thought stopping:** where an alternative thought has been prepared and can be triggered by a cue, such as a loose rubber band being flicked to catch the person's attention and access the alternative thought.

Relapse prevention

Having established a trusting and supportive therapeutic rapport the person may feel able to disclose thoughts that they might have otherwise feared sharing should they recur in the future. Through developing, practising and using these techniques the person will be able to independently manage intrusive thoughts and avoid the distress these cause. They may then feel more confident and competent in managing their mental health and through understanding the rationales for these interventions develop other additional methods that might be used.

References

Institute of Psychiatry, Psychology and Neuroscience (2014) Paranoia, www.mentalhealthcare.org.uk/paranoia, accessed 22 October 2014.

Sound-Mind.Org (2013) Obsessive thinking: ending scary thoughts, www.sound-mind.org/obsessive-thinking.html, accessed 31 October 2014.

Further reading

Clark, D.A. (ed.) (2005) *Intrusive thoughts in clinical disorders: theory, research and treatment.* New York: The Guilford Press.

Coleman, R. (2011) *Recovery: an alien concept,* 3rd edn. Inverness: P&P Publishing.

Romme, M. and Escher, S. (2015) Exploring the meaning of voices, www.intervoiceonline.org/tag/romme-and-escher, accessed 17 April 2015.

Negative thoughts

Definition/context

Negative thoughts are unfavourable understandings of situations and share the characteristic that they are plausible and credible but also have a number of other features. Among these are that they:

- are unwanted
- can be believed
- focus on negative aspects
- make the person feel bad
- represent a biased view.

(Resilient Mindset, 2012)

There are a range of common thinking styles in which negative thoughts are apparent (see Appendix 2 at the end of this chapter). Everyone experiences negative thoughts and these can take a wide variety of different forms, and represent a problem when they influence how we feel, think and behave.

Engagement

On initially meeting with the person their negative thoughts might be quite readily apparent in the form of repeated phrases, themes or ideas. However it is advisable to focus instead on understanding the person, building trust and demonstrating empathy. You should avoid challenging the negative thoughts directly until a therapeutic rapport has been developed with the person. This is because, in many cases, even where the person is aware of the negative thoughts, they nevertheless seem to have persuasive value and the person may need support over time to develop the confidence and resolve to challenge them.

Assessment

In assessment it is useful to help the person identify what is the 'hot thought'. Such thoughts tend to be very powerful, or trigger particular feelings, and so are generally easy for the person to recognize. The mental health nurse might also ask the person to encapsulate what they understand to be the content of the hot thought in a statement.

For example, the person may describe their feelings of self-doubt as: 'You can't possibly achieve that.' In this way we may accurately capture the person's description and understanding of the nature of the thought. However, it also allows the person to reflect upon the emotional impact of the hot thought. This can further be clarified by, for example, using a rating scale of believability of the thought from 0–10 with 0 being the lowest and 10 the highest. By rating the thought a baseline measure can be set against which to measure future improvement and therapeutic progress.

Care planning

In discussing the planning of care it helps to consider what the person wants to change and how their life might be improved. If the person can identify the benefits of no longer experiencing the negative thought, this might help them feel motivated to change and participate in interventions. However, in some cases the person may need to be facilitated to realize the effects of negative thoughts on their mood.

Intervention

In some cases by this stage the person has already recognized the 'hot thought', and has understood the effects of this on their feelings and behaviour, and formulated it into a statement. Using diagrams can help to make these connections more clear. A 'vicious cycle' can be drawn to illustrate links between thoughts, feelings and behaviours and to show how recurrent negative thoughts can keep a such a cycle going.

In some cases the person may have not recognized the effects of the negative thought. To help them to do this, the mental health nurse may ask very brief and focused questions that will help the person understand the connections between their thoughts and mood. So for example in response to the thought, 'You can't possibly achieve that' I may then experience feelings of doubt and self-blame or uncertainty and avoid carrying out challenging tasks.

It is also possible that in response to recognizing the negative thought and the detrimental effect that this has upon my feelings I can appreciate the negative thought as just one way of viewing the situation, and appreciate that there are other alternative perspectives that might be equally or more valid and produce a better impact on my feelings and hence a more advantageous outcome. Therefore I might build an alternative thought with which to challenge the negative thought (cognitive restructuring). So, for example in response to the thought: 'You can't possibly achieve that' a contrasting view would be, 'In the past I have achieved that, and more besides.' By identifying the person's rating of the thought in terms of strength of belief from 0–10 we can measure how effective we have been in challenging the negative thought. It may take time to embed this new thought, however patience in establishing the thought may lead to it being more effective in the longer term and building the person's confidence.

Relapse prevention

It will help to encourage the person to actively monitor their thoughts on an ongoing basis, in order to identify the recurrence of negative thoughts, or the emergence of new forms of negative thought. Practising reflection on thoughts and using the same methods and techniques that have been learned in working with thoughts that are unhelpful will continue to ensure positive mental health and well-being.

References

Resilient Mindset (2012) Negative automatic thoughts, www.resilient-mindset.com/2012/10/22/negative-automatic-thought, accessed 16 October 2014.

Further reading

Cognitive Behaviour Therapy Self-Help Resources (2014) About automatic thoughts, www.getself-help.co.uk/thoughts.htm, accessed 16 October 2014.

Appendix 1: types of delusion

Type of delusion	Example
Bizarre	Charles VI of France believed he was made of glass
Depressive	The person believes, contrary to evidence, that they have a serious illness
Erotic	Thinks that another person is in love with them
Grandiose	Believes they have special powers
Jealous	Thinking that their partner is having an affair
Nihilistic	The belief that the person, or world, has ceased to exist
Persecutory	Harm is going to happen that is intentionally inflicted
Religious	Believes they are a famous religious figure
Somatic	Thinking their body has been altered

Appendix 2: negative thinking styles

Thinking style	Example
All-or-nothing	If I don't do it right, then I'm useless
Catastrophizing	If I don't pass the exam, then I'll end up destitute and homeless
Negative bias	Bad things always happen to me
Perfectionist	I can't stand it if my house doesn't look absolutely pristine for visitors
Personalization	Although I won player of the match my team lost – it's my fault
Prophetic	If I say I can't do the favour, then she won't like me any more

13 Feelings in mental health

Feelings are the state of our emotions at any particular time, in other words, our mood. Often we are unaware of just how influential these are upon how we think and behave. In this chapter we will consider five aspects of mood: anger, anxiety, elation/excitability, lack of feeling and sadness.

Anger

Definition/context

In life there are many experiences that lead us to become angry, ranging from resentment and feeling let down in a specific situation, to a response to a perceived injustice or a gradual and growing feeling over a prolonged period – for example, of not being appreciated in your job or a relationship. Experiencing and expressing these feelings is a necessary part of interacting, living alongside and having healthy relationships with other people. In most cases these feelings are managed and mediated in our relationships and interactions with others. However, for some people anger is a problem, and they may express these feelings disproportionately to the situation, through destructive actions or behaviour towards others, or respond in a way that they later regret and wish they had acted differently.

One understanding of anger is as a response to a challenge that is perceived as potentially threatening or harmful (Mental Health Foundation, 2014). Anger and anxiety are linked through being contrasting responses to the 'fight or flight' instinct. In the case of anger, when comprehending a threat the body produces adrenaline which creates a state of heightened stimulation in preparation to act (Cognitive Behaviour Therapy Self Help-Resources, undated; Psychologistworld, 2015). This response is thought to be due to our long distant past and is engaged in order to protect us against physical threats and challenges. However, in modern life and our often much safer environment, the less directly life-threatening challenges that we encounter mean this sometimes produces unwanted or unhelpful outcomes. Often problems with anger occur where we misinterpret threat signals and react angrily, where instead another choice of action is more appropriate, or would produce a better outcome.

Often, though not exclusively, anger that is experienced as a problem is caused by abuse (emotional, physical, psychological or sexual), assault or traumatic experiences, though it may also be due to neglect, or emotional abandonment. People who experience post-traumatic stress disorder (PTSD) or personality disorder may express anger inappropriately and this can make it difficult for them to form relationships, and be very distressing for the sufferer and for those who are close to them.

Anger can also vary in intensity between individuals and is expressed in different ways (see Appendix 1 at the end of this chapter). For example, some people may be prone to impetuous or unpredictable behaviour, while others struggle to articulate how they feel, so it builds up and is eventually expressed through explosive outbursts. Anger can also be caused by difficulties in being assertive, a lack of social skills and feeling disempowered (see aggressive behaviour, Chapter 11, pp. 101–3). In these cases it may become evident through negative comments, avoidance and unspoken resentment towards the person who is the source of the anger, or the person who is angry turning their feelings inwards in the form of self-harm.

Engagement

Often our feelings are difficult to control or understand, and the person may not be aware of the effect of their anger on others, except that it produces negative responses and may cause problems for the person in their work, social life and close relationships. Therefore they may be aware of experiencing a problem but not really understand it and feel guilty or ashamed, yet also powerless. To help the person feel in control of their care it may help to begin by engaging in some preliminary discussion in general terms about what they may wish to change or improve in their life and asking the person what they perceive to be the problem.

Assessment

It is necessary to identify the nature and frequency of the person's anger, and how it arises in specific situations, using the 4WFINDSs approach (Skinner and Wrycraft, 2014).

What form did the anger take? Was there conflict with another person, was it expressed indirectly, or not expressed at all? Were the feelings of anger strong at the time yet dissipated through being expressed, for example after an argument? Or is there perhaps a lasting and residual sense of resentment directed against the person causing the anger, if it was not expressed?

Care planning

Care planning ought to be organized in three stages:

- first recognizing the situations in which the person becomes angry
- second, coming to an understanding of the link between feelings and behaviours, supporting the person to disrupt their anger in response to the felt emotion
- finally, helping the person to form more constructive and considered alternative responses to anger-provoking situations.

Intervention

Often due to the immediacy by which we are affected by moods, the connection between experiencing the feeling and acting can seem instantaneous and hard to disrupt. It will help to reassure the person about this, for example by acknowledging that we all behave and act in ways that we might regret at times but that we can still learn to respond differently.

It will help to assist the person to be able to:

- explain who or what is causing the anger
- identify what they feel would have improved the outcome of the situation.

In a safe environment and from a reflective perspective, the person can begin to appreciate the connection between their feelings and behaviours that at the time seem instantaneous. It is then possible to devise other alternatives that they might choose in similar situations in the future and to then practise these in their life in order to feel confident using them.

Among the measures that might be used to disrupt acting on the basis of feelings of anger are:

- breathing techniques
- deliberately delaying before reacting, for example counting to 10
- relaxation techniques.

(Mind, 2014)

It might also be useful to listen to music or to think about a calming song. Engaging in self-talk in response to the feeling might also reduce its intensity, for example, rationalizing the situation in a way that explains the anger or thinking: 'I'd love to say this to you . . .', but not actually saying it.

In cases where anger is not expressed or directed inward because the person feels disempowered or unable to outwardly demonstrate their emotion, it will help to focus on building assertiveness skills. This may be achieved through role play or behavioural experiments in situations that are identified as challenging but where the person feels able to attempt a new behaviour and then reflect on the outcome.

In addition to this, anger may be addressed by the following physically focused health considerations:

- diet
- exercise
- sleep
- life stress.

(Mind, 2014)

Relapse prevention

Central to maintaining change is learning new habits, and achieving competence in appraising threatening situations and in the skills and coping mechanisms used in challenging situations. Therefore practice is needed and perhaps the support offered by intermittent contact with a mental health nurse to help reinforce this new learning. Furthermore, it is important to exercise self-compassion, accept that we will not always get it right all of the time, and be prepared to learn from mistakes. It is also worth being aware that change is always possible. While this notion implies that we can avoid getting caught in a cycle of repetitive maladaptive behaviour, it is also the case that we need to continue to work at maintaining positive change.

References

Cognitive Behaviour Therapy Self Help-Resources (undated) Anger, www.get.gg/anger.htm, accessed 18 November 2014.

Mental Health Foundation (MHF) (2014) Anger, www.mentalhealth.org.uk/help-information/mental-health-a-z/A/anger, accessed 25 October 2014.

Mind (2014) How to deal with anger, www.mind.org.uk/media/42890/how_to_deal_with_anger_2012.pdf, accessed 25 October 2014.

Psychologistworld (2015) Stress: fight or flight response, http://psychologistworld.com/stress/fight-flight.php, accessed 20 January 2015.

Skinner, V. and Wrycraft, N. (2014) *CBT fundamentals: theory and cases*. Maidenhead: Open University Press.

Anxiety

Definition/context

Anxiety is a feeling of persistent agitation or restlessness over a prolonged period of time and another response to the 'fight or flight' instinct (see anger, above p. 126).

While in some cases, such as phobias, the person's anxiety may pertain to specific things or situations, in contrast, with generalized anxiety disorder (GAD), there is not necessarily any specific issue that triggers the anxiety at any particular time and the source of the problem may change. GAD is a frequently experienced mental health issue. However, anxiety is also present in other conditions, such as obsessive compulsive disorder (OCD), phobias and post-traumatic stress disorder (PTSD). Anxiety is also commonly experienced with depression and is an element of many other mental health issues. There are a range of bio-psychosocial features of anxiety (see Appendix 2 at the end of this chapter). Often anxiety is experienced as anxious feelings, for example of being out of control, unable to influence events, being in a state of panic, or being fearful of events. This then feeds into negative thinking or expectations from situations, and in turn influences the person's behaviour, forming a vicious cycle.

Engagement

People who are anxious may often feel that things are happening very quickly and have difficulty concentrating and focusing on what is being said to them. Therefore it helps to capture the person's focus, by, for example:

- keeping questions and comments brief
- maintaining close, though not intrusive, eye contact
- offering regular summaries of issues that are discussed
- regularly checking the person is following the conversation
- speaking clearly.

Assessment

There are a wide range of features of anxiety that affect people behaviourally, physically, cognitively and emotionally (see Appendix 2). In assessment it is necessary to consider how these differing elements act in combination to influence the person's behaviour, and to focus on the nature, scope and intensity of anxiety that the person is experiencing, using the 4WFINDSs (Skinner and Wrycraft, 2014).

Care planning

How we feel is often very persuasive and frequently goes unquestioned. The manner in which a person's thoughts and behaviours unhelpfully influence their feelings and cause problems may be very clear to the mental health nurse but much less evident to the person. Therefore, it is helpful to patiently explain the connections between thoughts, behaviours and feelings, and wherever possible allow the person to discover these for themselves in order to empower their learning and promote self-discovery.

This is especially important because anxiety can often lead the person to be indecisive or defer to others. If planning care is to be successful it is necessary that the emphasis is on supporting the person to determine their own choices wherever possible. Although there ought to be an emphasis on collaboration and partnership working, the more the process of care planning and the priorities chosen reflect the service user's preferences and choices, the more likely that process is to be successful.

Intervention

As is often the case with mood-related mental health problems it is necessary to facilitate the person in recognizing the triggers and symptoms of anxiety as they emerge. When working with the person it will help to develop and strengthen their skills when placed in anxiety-provoking situations. As with anger, and in common with mood-led disorders, the emphasis ought to be on reducing the person's need to respond to the immediate stimulus, commonly referred to as 'exposure response prevention' (ERP) (Skinner and Wrycraft, 2014). In ERP the person places themselves in a feared situation and resists their anxious fears while remaining in the situation. Through negotiation the person may identify a situation that on the one hand provokes anxiety but on the other is one that that they feel they can confront. Therefore, in discussing the planned exposure it will help to establish a hierarchy of feared events that may form a series of ERP experiments (Skinner and Wrycraft, 2014). Then, outside the session, the person places themselves in the situation but does not act on their fear, having already identified their anxiety level before exposure to the feared situation (see Appendix 3 at the end of this chapter). Reflecting on the experience afterwards allows the person to better understand their response but also to realize how managing in these fear-provoking circumstances builds their confidence, and contributes to how they might appraise the same situation differently in the future.

Other measures that might be used for a person with anxiety include:

- challenging negative thoughts by identifying evidence to prove or disprove their content
- practising progressive muscle relaxation, and following a scripted exercise to reduce the physical effects of anxiety
- practising relaxation techniques, including imagery and controlled breathing together with progressive muscle relaxation
- keeping thought records, to identify the connections between these and feelings and behaviours in the person's daily life
- keeping mood charts, to monitor periods where the person's mood influences how they think and behave
- recognizing cognitive distortions, or tendencies to think in ways that exaggerate expectations from situations
- practising mindfulness and meditation.

(Therapist Aid, 2014)

Relapse prevention

It is necessary to strike a balance and exercise careful judgement in allowing the person to cope independently with the intention of them gaining confidence through coping and offering support. In order to reduce the possibility of relapse it is necessary to check that the person's ability to cope is sufficiently adaptable to respond to a reasonable range of challenges. As time goes by, these skills can even be used to apply to different problems to those with which the person originally presented.

References

Skinner, V. and Wrycraft, N. (2014) *CBT fundamentals: theory and cases*. Maidenhead: Open University Press.
Therapist Aid (2014) Therapy worksheets related to anxiety for adults, www.therapistaid.com/therapy-worksheets/anxiety/adults/1, accessed 2 December 2014.

Further reading

Cherry, K. (2014) Generalized anxiety disorder – symptoms and treatments, http://psychology.about.com/od/psychiatricdisorders/a/genanxietydis.htm?utm_term=anxiety%20psychology&utm_content=p1-main-1-title&utm_medium=sem&utm_source=msn&utm_campaign=adid-6e1b913a-c158-4816-af65-3b3a56a60eb5-0-ab_msb_ocode-4343&ad=semD&an=msn_s&am=broad&q=anxiety%20psychology&dqi=anxiety%2BWorksheets%2C%2BHandouts%2C%2BResources-%2Band%2BTechniques%2B%2BPsychology%2BTools&o=4343&l=sem&qsrc=999&askid=6e-1b913a-c158-4816-af65-3b3a56a60eb5-0-ab_msb, accessed 19 November 2014.
PsychologyTools (undated) Anxiety, http://psychology.tools/Anxiety.html, accessed 19 November 2014.

Elation/excitability

Definition/context

Elation can be understood as when a person's mood is elevated beyond their normal range for a prolonged period, and is often evident as a disproportionate or inappropriate response to events. Due to their raised mood the person may appear very animated or flamboyant in mood, manner and response, and perhaps prone to behave spontaneously and impetuously. Often elation or excitability is a feature of bipolar disorder or psychotic illness.

Among the physical health-related factors that might lead to elation or excitability are:

- use of alcohol or caffeine
- use of illicit drugs or substances
- experiencing a traumatic incident or event
- hormonal issues
- physical ill-health
- sleep deprivation.

(GoodTherapy.org, undated)

Engagement

Often people with an elated mood are easy to engage, as they may have a keen and intense wish to share their feelings with other people. Yet they may also struggle with turn-taking, focusing on specific topics of conversation, and may monopolize the discussion, due to everything happening very quickly and feeling a need to urgently share information (see turn-taking, Chapter 3, pp. 28–9). Furthermore, the pace of the person's thoughts and speech may be rapid and lacking logical sequence or coherence. This can have the unhelpful effect of spiralling, leading to the person becoming confused and distressed and difficult to engage. Therefore it may help at the outset to identify ground rules and boundaries. For example, emphasizing that while there will be time for each party to express their views:

- the conversation will involve turn-taking
- each person will listen to the other
- there is a mutually agreed agenda
- the meeting will have a specific duration.

Furthermore, it may be helpful for the mental health nurse to use interpersonal skills, for example offering regular feedback, seeking clarification and summarizing what has been discussed to help structure and pace the conversation (see Chapter 3).

Assessment

In the mental health nursing assessment it will help to gain an understanding of the problem by establishing the extent, nature and frequency of the person's elation and excitability. This may be identified through discussing the issues about which the person is concerned and using a loosely structured type of assessment (see Chapter 1, p. 9). The reason for this is that attempting a formal and very structured assessment may be too rigid, whereas being flexible will incorporate the person's frame of mind and mood, yet allow for the fact that they may at times stray from the focus of the conversation. This represents a person-centred approach, and prevents the process feeling awkward and potentially undermining the therapeutic rapport.

The person's capacity to be able to provide an accurate account of their experience may be patchy and incomplete, differ from other people's accounts, or even by their own admission be unreliable. Often in states of elevated emotion it is difficult to provide a factual and objectively accurate account. Therefore it may help to ask the person to keep a record of how they experience events in the future, either on structured recording sheets or in a journal, and to monitor their mood. This information can later be reviewed and will form an important part of the assessment and subsequent planning of care.

Care planning

In planning care with the person it will help to maintain the positive and collaborative working rapport established in engagement and assessment, and also to be aware of the need to be clear, consistent and reliable in approach and in the interventions that are agreed. This is because the nature of this problem means that the person may be prone to mistrusting their perceptions, and may frequently feel a sense of flux. They will therefore benefit from a therapeutic approach that offers stability and consistency. Furthermore, this will promote trust in the therapeutic rapport and process if the person's mental health worsens, or they experience adverse life events (GoodTherapy.org, undated). Therefore, care planning needs to be carried out with an awareness of long-term goals that are achieved over time.

The information from the assessment and the person's journal can be reviewed and discussed. It will be possible to identify any patterns that are evident and it may help for them to see the problem from this objective vantage point, and with the support of the mental health nurse make sense of feelings that may be confusing or distressing.

Being able to review situations that have already happened allows the person to contemplate other possible choices of response that might have been taken and consider alternatives that could be carried out as interventions.

Intervention

Where the person experiences a constant feeling of elation they may need to see a doctor, with a view to possibly being prescribed medication to stabilize their mood before engaging in psychologically focused work.

If the problem is in relation to certain specific events or people, then it is possible to consider what it is about the person's thoughts that in certain situations leads them to respond differently than in other situations, where their mood is not altered. From this basis they may then consider alternative thoughts that make sense of the situation and do not trigger an excited mood, and then practise inserting these into the scenario. This may require role play and behavioural rehearsal, or carrying out behavioural experiments in their daily life in order to embed these ideas within their thinking and build a wider range of accessible feelings. Through handling situations better the person may also feel more confident and adept at handling issues which will add to their proficiency in managing their emotions.

Relapse prevention

Continuing to practise methods of appraising situations will help the person make a sustained improvement. Therefore, working with the person at their own preferred pace throughout the process, and ensuring that everything is explained clearly and makes sense to the person, will effectively ingrain good habits, and achieve better long-term sustainable results.

Due to the potential for the problem to spiral once it becomes apparent, it is necessary to:

- have a relapse prevention plan that identifies features when a relapse is likely
- be aware of who to contact (by name) in the event of a relapse
- for this information to be shared between all of the people involved with the person's care
- for actions to be identified to take in the event of a relapse
- to be aware of how it will be known when the problem has been resolved.

It is also helpful to ensure that the person takes any prescribed medication and that they understand the intended action and detrimental effects of not taking it as prescribed. It is also necessary that this is periodically reviewed and checked, either by the mental health services or the person's GP.

References

GoodTherapy.org (undated) Mood swings, www.goodtherapy.org/therapy-for-mood-swings.html, accessed 19 November 2014.

Further reading

34 Menopause Symptoms (2014) Mood swings, www.34-menopause-symptoms.com/mood-swings. htm, accessed 1 May 2015.
Krull, E. (undated) Mood swings are exhausting, http://psychcentral.com/blog/archives/2009/01/29/ mood-swings-are-exhausting, accessed 19 November 2014.

Lack of feeling

Definition/context

Lack of feeling refers to the loss of usual emotional content in situations and the ability to enjoy experiences. For example, a person may be watching their favourite programme on the television and following the storyline but not feel any emotional engagement. In everyday life the person may also feel that they are present at events but not really there. If this occurs over a period of time the person may feel that a significant amount of time in their life has simply not happened because it has left a very limited emotional impression upon them. Often lack of feeling is experienced as a feature of depression.

Engagement

The person may appear withdrawn and flat in mood, and attempts to engage them in conversation will be met with a very limited verbal and non-verbal response and interpersonal engagement. Initially it may help to make observations about the kind of day it is, to ascertain the person's response. If successful this might be developed further by asking brief and simple questions, perhaps of a neutral nature, that might establish a working rapport and demonstrate an interest in the person, but allow for an open response, for example, 'How is your mood today?' or 'Can you describe how you feel?'. It may also be the case that there is a delay between asking questions and gaining a response because of the person's low mood or lack of energy. Being patient, continuing to be positive in interpersonal and non-verbal communication and waiting for the person's response acknowledges their need and demonstrates an interest in their viewpoint.

Assessment

It may help to use a structured assessment that provides a format and logical sequence for the discussion. This is because lack of feeling is frequently accompanied by other features of depression, such as loss of motivation that may make the spontaneity of thought required for informal interviewing difficult, and a formal interview easier. Furthermore, a structured, formal assessment will allow for logical and natural collection of the information (see Chapter 1, pp. 8–9). It is possible that seeing the situation in this light might make the problem clearly evident, both to the mental health nurse and the person experiencing the problem. The information that will be collected will include the 4WFINDSs approach (Skinner and Wrycraft, 2014) along with information about:

- how long the person has experienced a lack of feeling
- in what situations the person notices and is aware that they lack feeling
- the thoughts they have about lacking feeling.

Due to their lack of feeling the person may not have consciously registered these aspects of functioning, and may have difficulty answering these questions. For example, in the case of a person who always watches a particular soap opera they may be aware that they are not enjoying life but not previously appreciated that they are not following the plot or enjoying watching the programme any more. Therefore it may be necessary for the person to monitor aspects of their life over a period of time before reporting back at a later date to appreciate the full extent of how their feelings have changed.

Care planning

Experiencing difficulty in feeling may lead the person to feel flat in mood, direction-less and hopeless. Therefore, in planning care, it will help to emphasize the forward-focused perspective of the working relationship and that the intention is to bring about change. However, to prevent the person feeling daunted it is important to also make clear that the therapeutic relationship will only progress at the pace at which the person wishes to work, and that it is founded on a basis of support and mutual regard.

The planning of care will build upon the assessment, and demonstrate to the person that over time they have felt differently, even if they were previously unaware of this. From this basis we can identify what it is that the person wants to change about how they are feeling, and how they think this might benefit their life and that of other people, for example significant others and family. In discussing the care planned interventions it will then help to taper down the discussion from general issues to consider particular themes that may form the basis of agreed interventions.

Intervention

Psychologically, it may also help to work with the person on the rationale that how we feel is often triggered by habituation, and in life we engage in some activities that we enjoy and others that we do not. How we respond to this is on a balance of enjoyment and endurance, yet a life that has balance includes a measure of each. Therefore, in planning care and seeking to reacquaint the person with experiencing pleasure it will help to negotiate activities in which they still find some enjoyment.

These can be identified using a graded hierarchy, with items listed ranging from those in which they find no pleasure to those in which they still experience some pleasure at times. The scale may be over a narrow range, with the person's pleasure rating initially still being quite low, yet with the aim of progressing in small steps. Between sessions the person then engages in activities they have identified as pro-ducing some pleasure and then rates the pleasure they felt. In this way the person may gradually improve their mood and begin to experience feelings of enjoyment again.

Additional interventions include seeking medical advice, and perhaps commenc-ing with antidepressant medication to lift feelings of pervasive low mood and address other features of depression that the person may be experiencing. However, it is worth bearing in mind that antidepressants often take some time to work, and there may be a delay between commencing medication and its taking effect.

Relapse prevention

In the long term the person should focus on continuing to sustain a balance between activities that are pleasurable and those that are less enjoyable. This work can be supported by planning daily activities and establishing routines to ensure that pleas-urable activities are a part of the person's daily pattern of activities. Follow-up ses-sions with mental health services to review progress will help to ensure that it has been maintained and to identify any further measures that are necessary. However, often a deterioration in mood occurs gradually and over time and it might help to agree with the person some markers whereby they are able to recognize that their mood is declining, and some measures to take to prevent further deterioration.

References

Skinner, V. and Wrycraft, N. (2014) *CBT fundamentals: theory and cases*. Maidenhead: Open University Press.

Further reading

netdoctor (2014) Anhedonia, www.netdoctor.co.uk/special_reports/depression/anhedonia.htm, accessed 19 November 2014.

Educational Portal (undated) What is anhedonia? Definition, treatment, symptoms and causes, http://education-portal.com/academy/lesson/what-is-anhedonia-definition-treatment-symptoms-causes.html#lesson, accessed 19 November 2014.

Sadness

Definition/context

Sadness becomes a problem where it is persistent and dominates a person's life, is in contrast with their normal character, and/or stops them functioning in their daily activities.

Sadness can be:

- a feature of depression among other factors
- a long lasting response to a loss or bereavement
- the result of a combination of detrimental life circumstances.

Through life people are sometimes prone to encountering detrimental or disadvantageous experiences that can lead to them experiencing sadness. However, in other cases there is no apparent precipitating factor.

Sadness can manifest in a variety of ways, for example:

- feeling inconsolable and sad over a prolonged period
- feeling that life is going slowly
- feeling pessimistic about the future
- feeling that life is negative
- feeling powerless
- feeling unable to participate in happy or positive events
- preoccupation with negative thoughts
- dwelling on specific unfortunate events
- tearfulness and expressing negative emotion.

Engagement

In engaging with the person experiencing sadness the mental health nurse will try and understand these feelings and empathize. However, as discussed in Chapter 3 (p. 25), while I may attempt to identify and empathize with another person, the best I can achieve is an approximation that can never adequately capture the personal experience of that feeling. Nevertheless, we can still try and learn from the person by asking them how their experience is affecting them. As discussed in Chapter 2 (p. 15), language and communication are shared mediums. While often language acts as a descriptor to convey information it is also a means of sharing what we think, our opinions and also how we feel. By sharing how we feel when distressed, the mental burden is reduced, even if nothing has actually happened to address the problem.

Assessment

With some people sadness may be readily evident through some, or all, of the features outlined above. However, the person's sadness may also be hard to detect. Outwardly they may appear to be completely unaffected, but inwardly they are experiencing profound turmoil and a deep-rooted sense of sadness. Some people are especially adept at appearing a certain way to others that masks how they really feel. It should never be assumed that because this is the case the person who is not self-evidently sad has less of a problem than the person for whom this is very clearly the case.

Establishing the four WFINDS of: What, Where, When and With whom (Skinner and Wrycraft, 2014) will clarify specific instances of problem, yet may allow the person to reflect on their feelings in the objective, safe and supportive context of the therapeutic rapport. It may be necessary to ask the person questions in different ways in order to elicit a response. If the first attempt at asking is not successful the mental health nurse ought not to feel that they have been unsuccessful or approached the situation well. Often assessment involves adapting the approach depending on what is learned from the person's response. In some cases words may be inadequate. Sometimes people feel more able to express their feelings in the form of images, visual representations or a cartoon character (Johnstone, 2007; Johnstone and Johnstone, 2008).

Care planning

In planning care it helps to focus on empowering the person and outlining the various therapeutic options that are available. It will help to adopt a person-centred approach where the pace is set in relation to the pace of the person, in order to demonstrate respect and appropriate consideration for feelings that are very important and intensely personal to the person. It may take time for the person to articulate how they feel, as often this can be quite elusive. If the person is experiencing other features of depression, their capacity to think, feel motivated and reflect on their situation and experiences may be affected.

It will also help to ascertain the person's level of motivation, as they may lack the desire to change and feel daunted at the prospect, and this in turn may hinder the pace of their treatment, and they may need to progress more slowly (see techniques of communicating in planning care, Chapter 5, pp. 43–5). It will help to collaboratively identify what the person wishes to achieve and change in their life.

Intervention

It may be necessary to seek medical advice and assess whether antidepressant medication may be suitable. Carrying out this intervention first is necessary, as antidepressants commonly take between two to four weeks to begin to work, and so the sooner the service user can start to take them then the more quickly they will gain the benefit. Furthermore, if the mental health nurse's contact with the service user is of a time-limited nature then they can offer support, advice and education on the effects as necessary when the person commences the medication.

The focus of psychological therapeutic work may be on other problems than the feelings of sadness. This will build trust and confidence in the therapeutic relationship, yet develop the person's problem-solving skills before considering the more challenging issue of their sadness.

Initially it may help to discuss the cognitive behavioural therapy (CBT) model and how our thoughts influence and impact upon how we feel and behave. The person will feel empowered by working with their thoughts to change how they feel. Positive thinking may be promoted by identifying and highlighting where the person has coped effectively before, and the skills and strengths this required. This is because often when experiencing low mood the person has a selective bias towards focusing on negative features at the expense of their positive skills. Introducing alternative thoughts highlights other possible perspectives for viewing situations.

It will also help to address repeated negative thoughts. This may take the form of monitoring thoughts to identify those that are negative. It is useful to encourage the person to engage in cognitive restructuring and identify an alternative thought to balance every negative thought that they experience (see negative thoughts, Chapter 12, pp. 123–5).

These methods may take time to establish, as negative thinking can become an established pattern. However, this is where the effectiveness of the therapeutic rapport becomes important, in the sense of investing a sense of trust and engagement in the therapeutic work.

For the person who lives alone, has limited social support or is bereaved, focusing on establishing routines and patterns to tasks in their life will help them remain active, while identifying social opportunities such as seeing friends, participating in leisure activities or taking up new activities, will also help. Particularly with regards to bereavement, it may help for the person to accept feelings of intense sadness and desolation in order to arrive at a new understanding and to have attended to feelings of grief and loss.

Relapse prevention

Sadness is a common human emotion that often has a gradual and pervasive onset. This can lead to the person losing interest in life and being caught up with and unable to disengage from their feelings. Yet learning and practising methods that work specifically for the person will help in building resilience and enhance their ability to cope.

References

Johnstone, M. (2007) *I had a black dog*. London: Constable & Robinson.
Johnstone, M. and Johnstone, A. (2008) *Living with a black dog*. London: Constable & Robinson.
Skinner, V. and Wrycraft, N. (2014) *CBT fundamentals: theory and cases*. Maidenhead: Open University Press.

Further reading

Kauffmann, J.C. (undated) Coping with grief, www.saga.co.uk/health/mind/coping-with-grief.aspx, accessed 20 November 2014.

Appendix 1: features of anger

The features of anger include the following.

Behavioural

- irritability or disagreeable manner
- foot tapping
- fist clenching
- aggressive or dominating body posture
- staring
- raised voice
- animated manner and gestures
- dramatic choices of words or swearing
- use of insults or personal remarks

Physical

- angry facial expression
- become flushed
- increased heartbeat
- rigid posture
- tightening of muscles

Cognitive

- 'all or nothing' thinking
- catastrophizing
- strongly adhering to own viewpoint
- seeing negative aspects of others' views

Emotional (feelings)

- confronted
- outraged
- undermined
- misunderstood
- tense
- offended
- upset

Appendix 2: features of anxiety

Anxiety has a wide range of features.

Behavioural

- excessive attention to apparently small or minor details
- irritability
- restlessness

- hypervigilance
- excessive levels of activity

Physical

- rapid breathing or breathlessness
- frequent urge to urinate, or experiencing diarrhoea
- sweatiness
- feeling hot
- feeling faint
- nausea
- sleeplessness
- knots or butterflies in the stomach
- exhaustion due to feeling anxious over a prolonged period of time
- muscular tension

Cognitive

- restless thoughts
- difficulty concentrating
- thinking that 'I'm going mad', or 'I can't cope'
- preoccupation with small or minor details
- experiencing events happening quickly

Emotional (feelings)

- fear or apprehension
- unable to meet demands
- mental fatigue/tiredness
- panic
- out of control
- unable to influence events
- upset.

Appendix 3: exposure response prevention (ERP)

Problem: social anxiety

Situation	Level of fear beforehand 0–10/10 with 0 lowest and 10 highest	Duration of exposure	Level of fear afterwards 0–10/10	Reflections
Being in a supermarket	6	55 minutes	3	Easier than I thought; waiting at the checkout was nerve-wracking

(continued)

Situation	Level of fear beforehand 0–10/10 with 0 lowest and 10 highest	Duration of exposure	Level of fear afterwards 0–10/10	Reflections
Asking for something specific in a shop	8	11 minutes	3	Was worried that they'd ask me questions about the item that I didn't know the answer to. Also when in the shop I felt anxious when there was a delay while the shop assistant looked up something on the computer but I kept my nerve
Phoning a friend I haven't seen in a while	7	17 minutes	2	I was very worried before, and not sure what to say, but afterwards was glad I made the call
Meeting the friend for a coffee	8	45 minutes	3	Was worried about dropping the cup and breaking it, and drawing attention to myself but dealt with this by being extra careful and it all worked out okay
Talking to a stranger about a minor issue	9	Not sure but very brief	2	Felt easy to do and will feel comfortable to do again

Case studies

14 | Case study 1: Jane

Jane is 34 years old. She has a very responsible job and often works long days into the evenings and is rarely able to take breaks for meals or rest. Recently during a meeting to discuss an important project Jane suddenly felt very hot, as though she was struggling for breath, became aware of her heart beating very rapidly and felt dizzy. On getting up to leave at the end of the meeting, Jane nearly lost her balance and felt as though she might pass out. Over the next few days she suddenly and unexpectedly experienced the same sensations again during meetings, and on the last occasion felt overwhelmed, as though the room was closing in on her, and passed out.

Jane's manager who was present suggested that she visit her GP, who carried out some physical tests that revealed no cause for concern. However, in discussion with the GP Jane became tearful and agitated and disclosed that she does not eat or sleep through preoccupation with work which dominates her life, and over time she has gradually felt more and more exhausted and low in mood. The GP signed Jane off work with exhaustion, and booked a follow-up appointment two weeks later to review her mood.

At the follow-up appointment the GP was concerned, as Jane looked as though she had lost weight, was dishevelled in appearance and seemed tired, low in mood and extremely agitated and tearful. Jane said she had seen no one since the last appointment with the GP and had not left her home due to feeling anxious. She was not eating and drinking and unable to sleep, and described feeling that she was a failure, that she was low in mood and fearful all of the time. When asked by the GP as to whether she had any plans to end her life Jane said that she did not want to live any more, although she had no active plans.

Assessment

The GP referred Jane to mental health services as an emergency. Initially the service felt Jane did not represent a high level of risk, as she did not seem to be a danger of violence or harm to herself or others. However the GP presented the view that Jane's self-neglect and living alone without social support meant there was the potential for her situation to very soon become a high-level risk to her physical health through self-neglect and also that her mental state might deteriorate further. The crisis resolution home treatment team (CRHTT) agreed to see Jane as a priority referral.

A community mental health nurse (CMHN) contacted Jane to arrange for an assessment. Jane was asked whether she would prefer to have the assessment at the team's office, or her home, and chose her home as she had recently felt reluctant to leave and described feeling uncomfortable visiting new places. Initially Jane was very quiet and subdued in the assessment meeting, saying that she was not sure what to expect as she had never been involved with mental health services. However, after some brief informal discussion she opened up, and seemed more comfortable. The CMHN used an informal style of assessment, with many open-ended questions (see Chapter 1, pp. 9–12).

Physical

Jane says she has always enjoyed very good physical health, and there are no issues with this regard in her family. However recently she experienced persistent colds, headaches and pains in her joints which she attributes to losing weight.

Eating and drinking

Jane appears very slight in build, and has not been eating or drinking, as she says she does not feel hungry or thirsty and forgets. Jane says that she takes no pleasure in food and finds eating to be a chore. She says she misses meal breaks in the daytime when at work and does not see the point in spending time to prepare food just for herself at home. She rarely goes food shopping and just has some basic staples in her home.

Self-care

Jane says that since not being at work she has lost her daily routine and often forgets to wash or carry out self-care as she knows that she will not see anyone in the daytime.

Sleep

Jane says she used to sleep well, however over the past few months has found sleeping to be a major problem. She describes herself as having no set pattern, and is often wide awake for long periods of time worrying, or has restless or fitful sleep and wakes up feeling tired.

Psychological

When growing up Jane says that her parents were focused on the academic performance of herself and her older brother and sister who are four and five years older than her respectively. As her siblings were much older than Jane but closer to each other in age she says they were closer to each other emotionally and describes always feeling like the odd one out. Jane describes being encouraged to be independent and self-sufficient from a young age by her parents and that they pointed out her older siblings as role models to aspire toward but Jane always felt she was 'not good enough'.

At school Jane doubted her ability and put in more effort than her classmates in order to achieve good grades, working through breaks and lunchtimes, missing leisure and after-school activities and then working in the evenings at home. While Jane was successful she says her parents were indifferent to this, which confirmed her own feelings of not being good enough. This, together with her being a very quiet and introverted person meant that Jane blended into the background and was not rewarded for her efforts in her schoolwork. She also found it very difficult to make friends at school, and later college, and often felt left out and rejected by her peers. Jane continues to feel: 'that I'm not as good as other people' and tends to make unfavourable comparisons.

Jane believes that her time off sick will count against her, that her employer might find another reason to dispense with her services, and that without her income she will not be able to afford her mortgage and will lose her home.

A risk assessment was carried out in the form of an open discussion with Jane about the nature of the risks. Jane and the CMHN felt that the care planned measures identified below were adequate to address and monitor Jane's risk of self-neglect. However, the CMHN also asked Jane whether she still felt that she did not want to live any more, as she had told the GP. Jane said that she still felt the same to some extent, although this had lessened. On a scale of 0–10 with 0 being the worst possible and 10 the best possible, Jane felt that her mood and sense of hopelessness when she saw the GP was a 2 but was now around a 3. Jane attributed this feeling to her low mood, yet also said she had no active plans to harm herself.

Sociological

Interests

Jane says that she does not really remember having many interests or hobbies when growing up, though she enjoyed reading and liked listening to music. As an adult she does remember enjoying going to the cinema to watch films, swimming and walking in the countryside. However, in recent times Jane says that she has stopped going out and become anxious about visiting new places, or anywhere that she does not know well. Jane says she wants to 'go places, maybe a coffee, and just enjoy myself and not worry'.

Relationships

Family

Her family only meet at Christmas, birthdays and some bank holidays. Jane feels that she does not get on well with her siblings and so does not have regular contact with them. However, she speaks regularly with her parents on the phone but does not feel that there is a close relationship with them. She has spoken with her parents since being off work but pretended everything was okay and did not tell them she was unwell, as she did not want to worry them.

Friends

Jane said she has no close friends, as although she made some good friends while at college she lost contact with them, explaining that work takes up most of her life.

Although spending a lot of time at work with colleagues that she likes as far as she is aware no one has contacted her, which Jane feels disappointed about. However, Jane has not been answering calls as she is unsure how to explain her absence if she receives any calls from her colleagues.

Significant others

Jane had a boyfriend until just over a year ago. The relationship lasted for four years, and at one point Jane thought they might marry and have children as she says that she dreamed of being a mother. However she discovered that he was seeing someone else and ended the relationship. They no longer have contact. In hindsight Jane says that she could see the relationship was deteriorating due to her commitment to work.

Care plans

Following the assessment Jane and the CMHN considered the range of her needs and discussed what the priorities were at this time, agreeing on the following care plans.

Physical need

Care plan 1: eating and drinking

Problem statement	Intervention actions	Date of review of the care plan	Outcome(s)	Date and signature
'I don't eat and drink regularly'	To be weighed initially to set a baseline measure and then to be weighed each week	Weekly	To increase my dietary and fluid intake and interest in food and maintain a suitable weight	dd/mm/yr Jane and the CMHN
	To plan what I will eat, and keep a food diary of three meals a day	Weekly		
	With my CMHN to look up recipes that I might like, and that I feel confident cooking and within my skill set	Weekly		
	To make a weekly shopping list	Weekly		
	To shop for food each week, initially accompanied by the CMHN	Weekly		
	To drink glasses of water regularly across the day and keep a diary of my intake	Weekly		

Care plan 2: sleep

Problem statement	Intervention actions	Date of review of the care plan	Outcome(s)	Date and signature
'I struggle to sleep at night and feel tired all of the time which affects how I feel'	Sleep hygiene techniques were discussed with Jane (see disturbed sleep pattern, Chapter 10, pp. 88–91). Jane has comfortable bedding and curtains with blackout blinds. Through discussion with the CMHN Jane agreed to: - 'wind down' and relax before bed, avoiding activities involving significant attention or stimulation - avoid caffeine or anything with stimulants in the evening - use relaxation methods, or listen to relaxing music before bed - have a regular bed time - have a bath or milky drink before bed. If unable to sleep to get up and engage in some 'low level' activity, such as reading, or listening to the radio - Jane also agreed to keep a sleep diary (see Appendix 1, Chapter 10, p. 100)	dd/mm/yr One month	For Jane to sleep better For Jane to feel more rested on waking For Jane's mood and sense of mental well-being to improve	dd/mm/yr Jane and the CMHN

Care plan 3: self-care

Problem statement	Intervention actions	Date of review of the care plan	Outcome(s)	Date and signature
'I would like to carry out my self-care, because I feel bad that I have let myself go'	To engage in activity scheduling and plan actions that I will carry out each day on a list, and tick them as I achieve them - Initially Jane will write activities on a post-it note, as the list will look less daunting - The activities will include self-care, beginning with washing her face and body - As Jane's confidence increases she will add to the list in discussion with the CMHN	dd/mm/yr Alternate days during visits with the CMHN	- For Jane to become more active, and have a structure to her day - For Jane to gradually carry out more of her self-care activities - For Jane to gain in self-confidence	dd/mm/yr Jane and the CMHN

Psychological need

Care plan 4: anxiety

Problem statement	Intervention actions	Date of review of the care plan	Outcome(s)	Date and signature
'I feel anxious all of the time, and would like to be able to relax'	Appointment with a psychiatrist, and possible prescription of antidepressant medication. - Support will then be given in terms of advice on any medication that is prescribed - Monitoring of any side effects - The medication will be discussed with Jane on a regular basis	dd/mm/yr Ongoing monitoring	To feel less anxious and more able to deal with anxiety	dd/mm/yr Jane and the CMHN

(continued)

Problem statement	Intervention actions	Date of review of the care plan	Outcome(s)	Date and signature
	Keep a mood diary, and monitor how I feel			
	For me to learn relaxation methods with the CMHN			
	For me to learn and practise techniques for relaxation to use when I feel particularly anxious. The CMHN agreed to discuss some techniques with Jane and identify some information that Jane can use	Ongoing		

Care plan 5: self-esteem

Problem statement	Intervention actions	Date of review of the care plan	Outcome(s)	Date and signature
'I believe that I'm not as good as other people'	In discussion with the CMHN for Jane to recognize negative thinking, the 'hot thought' (see Chapter 12, pp. 123–5) For Jane to consider the effect of the 'hot thought' on how she feels For Jane to develop and practise other positive thoughts that counter the 'hot thought' For Jane to engage in self-compassion when experiencing negative thoughts. For example, by asking herself, 'If a friend told me they were thinking this, what would I say?'	dd/mm/yr Weekly	To identify negative thinking and challenge these with more positive thoughts that produce a more beneficial outcome	dd/mm/yr Jane and the CMHN

Care plan 6: risk

Problem statement	Intervention	Date of review of the care plan	Outcome(s)	Date and signature
Jane has said that she does not want to live any more, although has no active plans	For the CMHN to monitor Jane's mood weekly during visits and activities to identify any indication of an intent to end her life, or plans to do so. Jane will continue to rate her mood each week using the 0–10 rating scale	dd/mm/yr	To monitor the possible risk of Jane ending her life on an ongoing basis	dd/mm/yr Jane and the CMHN
	For the CMHN to identify any significant changes in mood or behaviour that may increase Jane's propensity to risk	Weekly	To identify changes in the level of risk as a result of Jane's mood	
	For the CMHN to identify any other emergent risk factors		To identify any other possible risks	
	Jane agreed that if she feels as though she will harm herself she will contact the CMHN or the crisis line		For Jane to take control of her own potential for risk	

Sociological need

Care plan 7: employment uncertainty

Problem statement	Intervention actions	Date of review of the care plan	Outcome(s)	Date and signature
'I worry about losing my job and experiencing financial problems'	For Jane to seek advice on employment situation and occupational health and discuss any concerns with the CMHN	dd/mm/yr	For Jane to feel less worried about work and challenge her thoughts	dd/mm/yr Jane and the CMHN
	For Jane to test her 'catastrophic' belief by using cognitive restructuring and identifying the factors that might support this belief, and those that might disprove the notion	Weekly		

Care plan 8: socialization

Problem statement	Intervention actions	Date of review of the care plan	Outcome(s)	Date and signature
'I would like to go places, maybe [for] a coffee, and just enjoy myself and not worry'	For Jane to go out to a café with the CMHN for a coffee, and to monitor how she feels before, during and after the coffee	dd/mm/yr Weekly	For Jane to develop social interests, confidence in social settings and to feel socially included	dd/mm/yr Jane and the CMHN
	Jane would like to learn and develop relaxation and mindfulness techniques that can be used to relax in social settings and to then self-monitor the use and effectiveness of these	As needed		
	Jane has agreed that it would help to identify activities that she might like to engage in and attend that fit with her interests and skills that she wants to develop in order to build confidence	On an ongoing basis with the CMHN		

15 Case study 2: Frank

Frank is 82 years old and has been married to Anna, who is 80, for 57 years. Frank enjoyed a long working career as a carpenter, while Anna worked as a nurse before they both retired. Over the next few years they explored different parts of the world, having many adventures and trips that they dreamt of when working. Frank and Anna have had a long and happy marriage and have two grown up sons, who between them have had three grandchildren that Frank and Anna enjoy seeing.

Since their grandchildren arrived Frank and Anna have led a quieter life, travelling much less and remaining largely in the locality of the small town where they have lived all their lives. However they have remained very active, working as volunteers at a local charity shop, helping with many community events and being enthusiastic members of a local walking group.

Recently Frank's best friend of many years experienced the unexpected loss of his wife due to an aggressive cancer and then shortly afterwards suddenly committed suicide. Following his death Frank also found out that his friend was in the early stages of dementia. Just after this there was a concern that Anna may have cancer. While tests proved to be unfounded Frank then experienced a fall while out walking and broke his hip.

Frank made a very good recovery physically, however he has been very reluctant to carry on with any of the activities he previously engaged in. He does not want to see people at all and seems to have lost motivation and interest in life.

Assessment

Anna persuaded Frank to see his GP who prescribed antidepressants. However Frank has always been sceptical of taking any medication and refuses to take them, saying that he does not want chemicals to make him feel a certain way. Yet Frank's mood continued to deteriorate, and so the GP referred Frank with his reluctant agreement to the mental health services and a CMHN made an appointment to visit Frank at his home. During some of the assessment the CMHN spoke with Frank and Anna but also separately with both Frank and Anna, in case there was anything that either of them wished to speak in confidence about.

Physical

Frank says that before his recent fall he has always enjoyed very good physical health and is a person who likes exercise and the outdoors. Frank feels reluctant to use medication of any kind.

Eating and drinking

Frank says that Anna does all of the cooking, and is a good cook and so he is never without anything to eat. Lately he admits to not taking any pleasure in food but is not sure if this is because he is using less energy due to not being so active, or his mood is lower, or both. Anna used to insist that they eat together at all mealtimes. However as Frank often stays in bed for a lot of the day he misses many meals. While not letting him eat in bed, Anna sometimes allows him to eat while sitting in his chair in the lounge.

Self-care

Frank used to have a routine and wash and shave each day. He also paid careful attention to his appearance. However in recent months he often does not shave or wash for several days or change clothes. Frank feels, 'I've let my standards slip and feel that I can't do what I used to.'

Sleep

Whereas Frank always used to get up early in the morning and be very positive and active, he now often stays in bed for much of the day. Frank is aware that this is counterproductive but feels unable to 'face the day'. When asked what he would like to do about this, Frank says, 'I'd like to get a grip and organize myself a bit better, so I have some sort of routine.'

He is not sure how long he sleeps each night but says he is awake often and for long periods of time and that, 'I'd just like to get a good rest so I don't feel tired all of the time.' Anna says that even though Frank is not restless she is aware of him being awake, and this has disrupted her own sleep pattern and affected her mood. Frank describes feeling tired constantly.

Psychological

Frank describes feeling guilty over the death of his friend and often thinking about the difficulties that he was experiencing before ending his life. Frank wishes he had done more to help and seen his friend more often, though he accepts that he was unaware of the difficulties he was facing. Frank says that he feels the weight of 'all these things going round in my head'. This, followed by Anna's 'health scare' and his own accident, suddenly made Frank acutely aware of his own vulnerability. He says that he feels that 'I have aged overnight' and feels 'stupid' not to have ever realized that he might be 'in this position'. Never having previously thought about his own mortality he now cannot stop thinking about it. Frank says that after all of the things that have happened recently he 'dwells on the bad things that have happened' and feels that other unfortunate events will occur.

However when asked whether he would ever contemplate suicide or hurting himself Frank seems surprised at the question and says, 'I just want to feel better.' He worries about the burden that his current low mood might be placing on his wife, saying, 'I feel that I make Anna miserable which is not what I want' and so he does not tell her how he feels.

Anna is extremely worried about Frank and unsure of how to help him. She says they used to talk all the time and about everything but now Frank does not speak to her. Anna has not addressed this with him as she was unsure if it was part of his low mood. Anna says that she feels 'shut out' and just wishes that she could help.

Sociological

Interests

Frank and Anna have always had a wide range of hobbies and interests, and been keen to learn new skills and engage in different activities. However in recent years they have stayed closer to home. Frank admits that following his recent accident he has 'totally lost confidence in doing things' and sees himself as very different from the previously skilled and capable person that he was, to the point that he is now 'scared to do any-thing'. When asked what he would hope for, Frank says 'I would like to occupy myself and gain satisfaction from doing things.' In terms of what activities this might involve Frank says, 'I would like to spend time and maybe do things with my grandchildren.'

Relationships

Family

Frank and Anna both came from what they describe as poor backgrounds. Anna's mother and father ran a small farm as tenants, and she describes remembering her early life growing up as 'a struggle to make ends meet' and that she was an only child as her parents could not afford to have any more children. Although she had a small family circle with few relatives, Anna says that she and her parents worked together and had a happy life. This made her really appreciate the things that she had and until now she and Frank have always worked as a team on any problem that they have encountered.

Frank's father worked as an electrician in a factory making speakers for audio equipment, while his mother worked at a launderette. Frank has a brother who lives in Australia and who he speaks to on the phone and his sons regularly Skype.

Friends

Frank describes himself as a quiet person, and his working life involved him spending a lot of time on his own. However together with Anna they have had a very active social life, with a range of friends from their different interests. Yet both Frank and Anna feel that in recent times this has changed and their social circle has reduced. Following Frank's recent low mood Anna says she is reluctant to make social arrange-ments due to concern at how Frank might cope. Frank says he loves seeing his grand-children. Recently he became tearful when one of his grandchildren visited which he describes as due to being 'overwhelmed by how happy his grandson made me feel'.

Significant others

Frank and Anna have enjoyed a long and happy marriage that they both describe fondly and are a devoted couple who describe each other as best friends who talk about every-thing. Until now they feel that they have not encountered any significant problems or setbacks in life. They describe very good relationships with both of their sons, who live close by with their own families, and with whom they have regular contact.

Care plans

Following the assessment the CMHN collaboratively discussed with Frank and Anna what might be suitable needs to focus on in planning care. The problem statements and interventions identified below were those that were prioritized. In some cases there is more than one problem statement, yet these were felt to refer to the same need, or a common theme.

Physical need

Care plan 1: self-care

Problem statement	Intervention actions	Date of review of the care plan	Outcome(s)	Date and signature
'I've let my standards slip and feel that I can't do what I used to'	I will make a list of self-care activities to do each day, and carry these out. For example: - shower once a day - shave each day - select new clothes from the wardrobe - comb my hair - check how I look in the mirror	dd/mm/yr Weekly	I would like to resume my self-caring activities	dd/mm/yr Frank and the CMHN

Care plan 2: sleep

Problem statement	Intervention actions	Date of review of the care plan	Outcome(s)	Date and signature
'I'd just like to get a good rest so I don't feel tired all of the time'	I will: - set an alarm before going to bed for a time that I want to get up in the morning - get up in the morning when my alarm goes - carry out activities in the daytime - set a regular time to go to bed The CMHN will discuss 'sleep hygiene' measures with Frank (see Chapter 10, p. 90) I will keep a sleep diary (see Appendix 1, Chapter 10, p. 100)	dd/mm/yr Weekly Weekly Weekly Weekly Weekly Weekly	I would like to establish a sleeping pattern that allows me to gain adequate rest	dd/mm/yr Frank and the CMHN

Psychological need

Care plan 3: feelings

Problem statement	Intervention actions	Date of review of the care plan	Outcome(s)	Date and signature
		dd/mm/yr		
'. . . all these things going round in my head'	I would like to meet with my CMHN each week, to talk about the things going round in my head	Weekly	I would like to feel less burdened by my thoughts and not so guilty about my friend	dd/mm/yr Frank and the CMHN
	Between sessions for Frank to reflect on how he feels about his life, and: - where he is at	Weekly		
	- his dreams, goals and aspirations	Weekly		
	To monitor how I am feeling on a regular basis, and to keep a diary of my mood writing down how I feel and rating my mood from 0–10 with 0 the lowest	Weekly	I want my mood to improve	
	To discuss with the CMHN how my low mood might affect how I think, feel and behave			
'Dwelling on the bad things that have happened'	To talk with my CMHN about my negative thoughts and consider the positives to balance my thinking, and help with how I feel	Weekly	To challenge my negative thoughts and realize how my thoughts influence my feelings and behaviour	

Care plan 4: mood

Problem statement	Intervention actions	Date of review of the care plan	Outcome(s)	Date and signature
'I feel that my mood might make Anna feel miserable which is not what I want'		dd/mm/yr	For Frank and Anna to communicate more effectively and to work together as a couple	dd/mm/yr Frank and the CMHN
	Frank and Anna will talk to each other every day about how he is feeling	Weekly		
	Frank and Anna will discuss what might help them both	Ongoing		
	Frank and Anna will carry out some activities together that they used to do before Frank's accident	Weekly		
	Anna will speak with the CMHN and multidisciplinary team to learn about how low mood affects people and receive support from the CMHN regarding her needs	As needed	For Anna's needs to be considered and for her to learn about how low mood may have affected Frank and how she might help him	Anna and the CMHN
	If required for Anna to talk to other people that have been carers for a person with low mood	If needed		

Sociological need

Care plan 5: socialization

Problem statement	Intervention actions	Date of review of the care plan	Outcome(s)	Date and signature
		dd/mm/yr		dd/mm/yr
				Frank and the CMHN
'I would like to occupy myself and gain satisfaction from doing things'	For Frank to consider activities that he might like to do and that he would gain satisfaction from	Weekly	I would like to begin to do things again and feel more confident	
'I would like to spend time and maybe do things with my grandchildren'	For Anna and Frank to invite their grandchildren over and spend some time with them	Weekly	I would like to spend time with my grandchildren	
	For Anna and Frank to meet up again and socialize with friends	Weekly		

Case study 3: Debbie

Debbie is 20 years old and lives with her mum and dad and two younger brothers aged 16 and 14. Debbie has experienced concern about her weight and often has feelings of anger towards other people. She identifies this as beginning when she was 14 and another girl began making insulting comments about Debbie's weight. This escalated when a number of other girls joined in and began taunting Debbie over a prolonged period of time. Debbie says that she 'eventually snapped' and attacked the girl who began it all, physically assaulting her, and as a result was excluded from school.

The incident was not in keeping with Debbie's nature. She is normally a quiet and considerate person and has never been involved in any other violent incidents. However since then Debbie has experienced thoughts that she is a bad person and unpopular with other people and that everyone is talking about her and looking at her. Debbie says that she is 'constantly running away from people' and 'can't deal with what they say'.

Debbie became very withdrawn, not speaking and avoiding other people wherever possible. At times she also became extremely angry with her parents and brothers over trivial or unimportant issues. Her parents originally felt that this was all a part of Debbie's adolescence and growing up. However Debbie has continued to isolate herself.

In spite of this Debbie trained as a beautician and hairdresser at which she is very skilled, building a good reputation and loyal client base. Debbie describes this as being useful in 'taking her out of herself' and helping her learn to value herself through care for her appearance. However Debbie is very self-critical of how she looks, her appearance and her diet.

Over recent months Debbie has experienced intrusive thoughts, particularly that she might harm people with her hairdressing scissors. These gradually increased in frequency and intensity, to the point that she feels that she can no longer work and is reluctant to leave home. Debbie often stays in bed all day, does not wash and will only eat reluctantly with prompting and encouragement. She does not want to speak to anyone. Debbie's GP made a referral to the mental health team.

Assessment

Debbie was contacted by a CMHN and expressed a preference to attend an assessment at the community team's office. She looked unkempt in appearance, was accompanied by her mum and initially seemed to be reluctant to speak, or engage in eye contact. Debbie said that she wanted her mum to be present at the assessment.

In the assessment the CMHN began with some informal questions, explaining how long the interview would last and that the information Debbie and her mum gave would be regarded as confidential but might be shared within the multidisciplinary team. The CMHN then explained that after the meeting there would be a discussion and then some suggestions as to measures that Debbie might find helpful in improving her mood and mental health.

Physical

Debbie experiences acute asthma and says that because of her work as a hairdresser she often has difficulties with breathing, and has frequent coughs and colds but otherwise has good physical health.

Eating and drinking

Debbie often only eats once a day in the early evening, and rigidly controls her dietary intake. She only eats certain types of food and avoids sweets, chocolate and anything that has a high fat content. Debbie reads all of the packaging and labelling on everything she eats and keeps track of the calorific content of the food she consumes. She says that her diet is boring and uninteresting. However when asked whether she might like to eat more varied and exotic food, Debbie says, 'I'd like to eat what I want but I put on weight much easier than other people.' Debbie believes that she is overweight and needs to carefully watch what she eats to avoid gaining weight. However at the assessment meeting Debbie was wearing loose-fitting clothing and seemed very slight in build. In spite of it being a warm day Debbie complained of feeling cold, even though she was wearing several layers of clothing. Debbie feels that her weight is unchanged recently but her mum says she thinks Debbie has lost weight recently. Debbie admits that she is not confident in her cooking skills, as her mum has always cooked for the family and she might like to begin to cook in order to gain independent skills and perhaps move out of home, but cannot afford it and can't ever imagine feeling able to cope.

Debbie admits that she does not drink as much fluid as she ought to and says it is because often drinks make her feel overfull or nauseous.

Self-care

Debbie says that she is particular about her appearance and looks after her self-care needs. However her mum says that until recently Debbie took much more care and interest in her appearance but lately seems to have lost 'pride in herself'.

Sleep

In the assessment Debbie said that although she has a generally settled sleep pattern, she sometimes thinks that if she relaxes or falls asleep she may be more prone to experiencing or even acting on her negative thoughts. However, in discussion Debbie remarked that she feels safe and comfortable sleeping in the bedroom that she has had since she was a child. The CMHN reflected back to Debbie that it is good to have things in life that provide security.

Psychological

Debbie says that she likes to feel in control of herself and this is why she restricts her dietary intake. Debbie experiences intrusive thoughts about harming people with her hairdressing scissors on a frequent basis. She says this happens without warning and she cannot 'switch them off'. Debbie feels very distressed by these thoughts because she says 'I don't know where they come from, it's as though they're not mine but I feel helpless' and that her thoughts are 'out of control'. Debbie worries that 'I'm going mad' and feels guilty and scared about the thoughts.

Debbie says she feels worried about the anger that she feels and so isolates herself from other people and particularly people she does not know well because of the possibility that she may become angry. Debbie says, 'I just wish I didn't feel so angry all of the time and could be calm like other people seem to be.'

Sociological

Debbie's mum describes the family as very quiet and 'keeping themselves to themselves'. They live in a very small house in close proximity to one another and do lots of things together. Debbie's mum says it is 'getting everyone down seeing how unhappy Debbie is all the time'. Debbie admits to feeling lonely and would like to see other people more and meet with friends and go out. When asked what she might like to do with her life Debbie says she would have liked to have taken more exams at school and feels that this would have given her more opportunities in life.

Interests

Debbie used to enjoy going to the gym on a regular basis several times a week until very recently but has stopped due to 'getting out of the habit' and 'losing confidence'. Debbie says she enjoyed going to the gym, swimming and going out with her friends but has lost confidence and does not see them any more out of fear that she may become angry and fear of her continuing intrusive thoughts, as she can never be sure when these will occur. However Debbie says, 'I miss enjoying myself and would like to see my friends again.'

Relationships

Family

Debbie is very close to her family and spends a lot of time with them. Debbie often carries out activities with her mum.

Friends

Although feeling suspicious of others after her problems at school Debbie has a few close and trusted long-term friends. However lately she has not wanted to meet with her friends and has not spoken to them recently. Debbie's parents are worried that she does not see other people and is becoming increasingly isolated and dwelling on her mood.

Significant others

Debbie has never been in a close relationship with another person, however she says that she would 'like to meet someone one day' but thinks it unlikely because she feels that she is 'fat and ugly'.

Care plans

After the assessment the CMHN met again with Debbie and her mum to clarify the priorities for her care plan.

Physical need

Care plan 1: diet

Problem statement	Intervention actions	Date of review of the care plan	Outcome(s)	Date and signature
		dd/mm/yr		dd/mm/yr
'I'd like to eat what I want but I put on weight much easier than other people'	- I would like to discuss with my CMHN my normal calorific intake, and how this compares with that for an adult female of my height and age	Ongoing	Debbie would like to eat a more varied diet and not put on weight	Debbie and the CMHN
	- I think it would help to look in more detail at my diet and agree to be referred to a dietician to look at whether I might eat a more varied and interesting diet	Ongoing		
	- I agree to be weighed to set a baseline measure that can be used to gauge any future changes. In order to avoid my becoming too focused on my weight it might be best to avoid regular or weekly weighing	Ongoing		
	- I agree to discuss hydration with the dietician and to drink water regularly throughout the day	Ongoing		
	- I would like to cook with my mum to gain confidence in the kitchen and learn skills		For Debbie to begin to develop independent cooking skills	
	- I would like to cook a meal for the family once a week	Weekly		
	- I would like to invite friends over for a meal that I have cooked	Future plan		

Psychological need

Care plan 2: anger

Problem statement	Intervention actions	Date of review of the care plan	Outcome(s)	Date and signature
'I just wish I didn't feel so angry all of the time and could be calm like other people seem to be'	I would like to discuss with the CMHN how anger works (see Chapter 13, pp. 126–129) and how my feelings influence how I think and behave - I agree to self-monitor my thoughts when experiencing anger - I think it will help me to develop coping mechanisms through discussing 'what works' with the CMHN - This care plan cross-references with care plan 3 (see below), as the source of this problem is in my past, and might be addressed by using revisualization	dd/mm/yr Weekly Ongoing Ongoing Ongoing	For Debbie to feel more in control of her anger and better able to manage her emotions	dd/mm/yr Debbie and the CMHN

Care plan 3: intrusive thoughts

Problem statement	Intervention actions	Date of review of the care plan	Outcome(s)	Date and signature
'I don't know where they come from, it's as though they're not mine but I feel helpless'	Consistent with Intrusive thoughts (see pp. 121–3) - I agree that it might help with support from the CMHN to revisualize the situation that caused the intrusive thought back at school when I was 14	dd/mm/yr At an agreed date once the rapport has been established Ongoing	I would like to feel a sense of control over my intrusive thoughts and gain confidence in dealing with them	dd/mm/yr Debbie and the CMHN

(continued)

Problem statement	Intervention actions	Date of review of the care plan	Outcome(s)	Date and signature
	- I think it will help to practise and then engage in positive 'self-talk' (see Chapter 12, p. 122) and reassurance	Ongoing		
	- It will help me to recognize the thoughts as negative 'self-talk', and to consciously turn down the volume; also to engage in 'thought stopping' (see Chapter 12, p. 122) and access alternative thoughts	Ongoing		
	- I agree an appointment will be made with my psychiatrist to discuss whether medication might help	Next week		

Sociological need

Care plan 4: social activity

Problem statement	Intervention actions	Date of review of the care plan	Outcome(s)	Date and signature
'I miss enjoying myself and would like to see my friends again'	- I think it will help me to contact a friend and arrange to meet with them	dd/mm/yr Next week	For Debbie to re-establish a social network and enjoy being with her friends	dd/mm/yr Debbie and the CMHN
	- I would like to meet with my friends on a regular basis to re-establish those close friendships	Ongoing		
	- I would like to discuss activities that my friends and I might like to carry out, for example going to the gym	Future plan		
	- I agree to discuss my progress with the CMHN	Weekly		

Care plan 5: carer's care plan

Problem statement	Intervention actions	Date of review of the care plan	Outcome(s)	Date and signature
To ascertain whether support is required for Debbie's mum, dad and brothers	- I agree for the CMHN to meet with mum and dad to discuss how my mental health affects them - I agree for the CMHN to provide my mum and dad with any general mental health information that might help them in supporting me - I think it helps that the CMHN is there to support my mum and dad in helping me - I agree that my mum and dad can contact the CMHN on their number or at their office in the event of a crisis - I agree for the CMHN to discuss the impact of my mental health on my brothers with mum and dad		To assess how Debbie's parents feel about her mental health, and to ascertain their needs To provide relevant education and information about mental health as needed To support Debbie's relationship with her parents To ensure that Debbie's parents are aware of a named mental health professional and their contact details in the event of Debbie experiencing a crisis To assess with the family the impact of Debbie's mental health upon her brothers and access further resources and support as needed	dd/mm/yr Debbie and the CMHN

Ade is 27 years old. His parents, Ade and his older brother who is now 31 moved to the UK when he was very young. When he was 11 Ade's mother committed suicide after a long period of depression. Ade describes living with his dad and brother as being 'very sad, because my dad struggled to cope and when we were together we were reminded mum wasn't there'. However when he was 15 his dad remarried and Ade and his brother went to live with his father, stepmother and her two children. Ade remembers this time fondly and he has a particularly close platonic relationship with his step-sister who is two years older than him and who he refers to as his 'big sis'.

Ade left home to go to university when he was 18 but found that he did not enjoy the course or university life. He began taking drugs: 'because I was feeling miserable, struggling with the work and didn't want to think about it'. On several occasions the police were called to the flat Ade shared with fellow students because of disruptive behaviour, or his playing loud music late at night. When he was 20 Ade was found wandering the streets in a confused state late at night and was taken to a mental health unit by the police under Section 136 of the Mental Health Act (1983, reviewed 2007). Ade was placed under Section 2 of the Mental Health Act for assessment and this was later amended to Section 3 for treatment.

While on the unit Ade reported hearing voices and one in particular that he said belonged to a medium who had contacted him and could bring his mother back. Ade said the voice was sometimes friendly but at other times could be unpleasant. It told him his mother died because of his sins and he had to atone for them. Ade's father and brother found the content of the voices offensive and this caused a rift in their relationship. Ade's inpatient admission lasted for some months as he did not believe that he was unwell and was resistant to taking medication or engaging in treatment.

When he was eventually discharged Ade went to live in a housing association flat and over the next 18 months had two further inpatient admissions, each time due to stopping his medication and rapidly becoming unwell.

Since then Ade has not relapsed for the last nine years and, while not in employment, has attended some further education courses and been supported in the community, regularly receiving visits from a CMHN to monitor his mood, mental health and well-being. Recently there have been several complaints about Ade playing music late at night, and he has been heard shouting out of the window and on one occasion was seen trying to stop traffic in the street. Ade's CMHN has noticed that he has seemed more agitated and lower in mood and has visited to carry out an assessment.

Assessment

On meeting the CMHN, in spite of knowing them well, Ade initially seemed agitated and a little preoccupied and anxious. On being asked about this Ade explained that he didn't 'want to go back in hospital again'. The CMHN explained that the meeting was to consider any changes to Ade's physical, psychological and sociological health for the purpose of reviewing his care plan and to identify any new measures that might help his mental health and well-being.

Physical

Ade has no known physical health issues, though he has regular check-ups regarding his physical health at his GP surgery. Ade smokes cigarettes and admits to using illicit drugs. He has been given advice and support about stopping smoking but has struggled as 'it is something to do and all my friends smoke which makes it hard to give up'. However Ade agreed to make an appointment with his GP practice to consider measures that might help him stop.

Eating and drinking

Ade appears to be a little overweight. He feels self-conscious about this, as he was always previously very slim and says he has gained weight in the last few years because he has not been so active. He says he would like to get 'back to being fit again'. Ade feels that he has also gained weight due to his having a limited food budget, as he is on benefits and so eats inexpensive processed food and ready meals. Ade would like to eat better and more healthily and to exercise so as to build a healthy appetite, but says he lacks the confidence and skills in knowing what to buy and how to cook different meals, or to go to a gym. Ade believes that budgeting better, gaining skills in cooking and doing some exercise would mean that he eats better, feels physically healthier and more alert and increases his confidence and how he feels about himself.

Self-care

Ade appeared reasonably well groomed, and was suitably dressed for the weather. He says he does not like washing clothes, so sometimes wears them for longer than he feels he should, but says he feels comfortable in them. He does not like cleaning the flat either, but though it was untidy it was clean, and when asked Ade said he felt it was clean enough.

Sleep

Ade says that he has been struggling to sleep lately and has had a disrupted pattern. When asked what might be causing this, Ade says that he feels low at the moment and generally anxious. Although Ade cannot think of a specific issue that has caused this concern the only significant change in his life recently has been that he has seen less of his step-sister. She used to visit him regularly but was not able to see him so often due to her having to travel and work away for more of the time, and he missed her. Ade says he would 'just like to get a good night's sleep'.

Psychological

Ade says that he is still taking his antipsychotic medication for the voices, even though he feels that 'it does not work'. This was discussed with the CMHN and the intended effect and action of the medication explained. Ade admitted that he does hear the voices less frequently and insistently when he takes it in comparison with when he does not. Ade feels that he would like to be 'more in control' of his illness.

When asked about his mood Ade said he has felt consistently lower in mood over the past few months and 'a bit down lots of the time'. Ade says he would 'like to feel a bit brighter and not quite so low'. When asked to rate his mood over the last two weeks from 0–10 with 0 the lowest and 10 as good as it could be Ade says he would score himself at the lowest 3 or 4 but at the best no higher than a 5. He says he often feels low when he is alone at home.

When asked if there was anything he would like to be different that would make him feel better Ade said that he would like to see his step-sister more frequently and was worried about losing touch with her, as she was the sole contact with his immediate family.

Sociological

Interests

In the past Ade often enjoyed reading science fiction books and doing word and number puzzles but has 'not done this for a while'. Yet when asked more about this Ade revealed that he has not been able to afford books or magazines. Ade also recalls that the further education courses he attended in the past were interesting.

Relationships

Family

Ade has not seen his dad or brother for several years. He feels that they have struggled to come to terms with his illness and misses them but hears about them through his step-sister. Ade feels guilty at their becoming estranged because of what he now accepts was his response to voices but at the same time feels like a victim of circumstance as he was ill. Ade admits that he often thinks about his dad and brother and would like to resume contact with them.

Friends

Ade is a sociable person and has several close friends that he meets with regularly and socializes with. In the past Ade had many friends and a wide social circle but felt that he was sometimes taken advantage of and persuaded to take drugs that did not help his mental health. Ade feels that he has 'grown up' and 'learned from my past mistakes'.

Significant others

Ade has had several girlfriends in the past but these relationships have never lasted. Ade says he would like to meet someone in the future.

Care plans

After the assessment the CMHN and Ade discussed what he regarded as his priorities and agreed the following care plans.

Physical need

Care plan 1: eating and drinking

Problem statement	Intervention actions	Date of review of the care plan	Outcome(s)	Date and signature
'I feel that I eat as well as I can but have a limited food budget due to being on benefits, so eat inexpensive processed food and ready meals'	- I think it will help for my CMHN to refer me to an occupational therapist to help me plan my food budget, shop with me and help me cook healthy meals - I would like to attend a cookery class held at a local day service and agree for my CMHN to make the arrangements	dd/mm/yr	Ade would like to eat more healthily within his budget	dd/mm/yr Ade and the CMHN

Care plan 2: exercise

Problem statement	Intervention actions	Date of review of the care plan	Outcome(s)	Date and signature
Ade would like to get 'back to being fit again'	- I will ask my GP for a referral to the gym, in order to develop a regular exercise programme	dd/mm/yr Within the next week	Ade would like to exercise so as to build a healthy appetite	dd/mm/yr Ade and the CMHN

Care plan 3: sleep

Problem statement	Intervention actions	Date of review of the care plan	Outcome(s)	Date and signature
Ade says he would 'just like to get a good night's sleep'	- The CMHN will discuss 'sleep hygiene' measures with Ade (see Chapter 10, p. 90) - Through increasing his activity in care plan 2 Ade may feel better able to sleep - I agree to keep a sleep diary (see Chapter 10, pp. 88–91)	dd/mm/yr Next week Over the next month to three months From next week	For Ade to establish a settled sleeping pattern	dd/mm/yr Ade and the CMHN

Care plan 4: smoking

Problem statement	Intervention actions	Date of review of the care plan	Outcome(s)	Date and signature
For Ade to consider measures that might help him stop smoking	- At the appointment with the GP (see care plan 2) I will ask about measures to help me give up smoking	dd/mm/yr Next week	Consistent with the above interventions, and as part of Ade's overall physical health plan to carry out measures that will improve his physical health and well-being	dd/mm/yr Ade and the CMHN

Psychological need

Care plan 5: medication

Problem statement	Intervention actions	Date of review of the care plan	Outcome(s)	Date and signature
Ade feels that his medication 'does not work'	- I agree for the CMHN to visit each week and discuss whether I have been taking it and how I feel about my medication - I agree for the CMHN to arrange a review of my medication and for there to be a meeting that the CMHN and I can attend together with the psychiatrist and multidisciplinary team	dd/mm/yr Each week Within a week	For Ade to continue to take his medication as prescribed and understand the intended action and positive effects	dd/mm/yr Ade and the CMHN

Care plan 6: mental state

Problem statement	Intervention actions	Date of review of the care plan	Outcome(s)	Date and signature
Ade would like to feel 'more in control' of his illness	- For Ade to make contact with the local Hearing Voices network and join a group - For Ade to develop methods and techniques that help him to live with the voices	dd/mm/yr Next week Within a week	For Ade to feel that he has control over the voices	dd/mm/yr Ade and the CMHN

Care plan 7: mood

Problem statement	Intervention actions	Date of review of the care plan	Outcome(s)	Date and signature
Ade feels 'a bit down'	- At the medication review with the psychiatrist for Ade's mood to be discussed and for it to be considered whether Ade would benefit from being prescribed antidepressant medication - For Ade to keep a mood diary (see Appendix 1) and, to rate his mood from 0–10 with 0 being the lowest and 10 the highest. Also to note the 4WFINDS of: When, Where, What and With whom (Skinner and Wrycraft, 2014) - Ade also agreed to monitor his thoughts and to keep a thought record (see Appendix 2) - For Ade's CMHN to discuss his mood diary and thought record with him each week	dd/mm/yr Next week Ongoing Ongoing Ongoing	Ade would 'like to feel a bit brighter and not quite so low'	dd/mm/yr Ade and the CMHN

Sociological need

Care plan 8: interests

Problem statement	Intervention actions	Date of review of the care plan	Outcome(s)	Date and signature
	dd/mm/yr	dd/mm/yr		dd/mm/yr
Ade used to enjoy reading science fiction books and doing word and number puzzles, also attending further education courses	- I would like to go to the local library and renew my membership - I would like to join a reading group at the library - I would like to begin a further education course at the local adult education college so will visit and get a prospectus and discuss courses that I might like to take with the staff and my CMHN	Over the next two weeks Over the next month Over the next three months	Ade would like to feel a bit more stimulated and involved in learning	Ade and the CMHN

Care plan 9: Concerns over step-sister

Problem statement	Intervention actions	Date of review of the care plan	Outcome(s)	Date and signature
		dd/mm/yr		dd/mm/yr
Ade is concerned about losing touch with his step-sister	- For Ade to talk with his step-sister about his fears - For the CMHN to support Ade as necessary and regularly seek feedback from Ade about his feelings and progress		For Ade to address his concerns over losing touch with his step-sister	

Care plan 10: Renewing family relationships

Problem statement	Intervention actions	Date of review of the care plan	Outcome(s)	Date and signature
	dd/mm/yr	dd/mm/yr		dd/mm/yr
Ade often thinks about his dad and brother and would like to resume contact with them	- Ade has agreed to talk to his step-sister about what he might say to his dad and brother - Ade will write a letter to his dad and brother and ask if they might meet with him - For the CMHN to support Ade during these interventions and regularly discuss his feelings about this and progress		For Ade to attempt to renew contact with his dad and brother	Ade and the CMHN

Appendix 1: Ade's mood diary

Date: –/–/—————

Time and activity	What?	When?	Where?	With whom?	Rating 0–10 How did you feel?

Appendix 2: thought diary

Date: –/–/————

Time and activity	What?	When?	Where?	With whom?	Rating 0–10 How did you feel?

Index

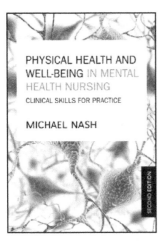

PHYSICAL HEALTH AND WELL-BEING IN MENTAL HEALTH NURSING
Clinical Skills for Practice
Second Edition

Michael Nash

ISBN: 9780335262861 (Paperback)
ebook: 9780335262878
2014

This popular and groundbreaking book was the first of its kind to focus on providing mental health nurses with the core knowledge of the physical health issues that they need for their work. Considering the risk factors and assessment priorities amongst different mental health client groups, the book provides clinical insights and current guidance into how best to work with service users to ensure their health is assessed and improved.

In this fully updated second edition the book addresses the current context and the latest research and policy, as well as expanding coverage of:

- **Assessment principles and skills**
- **Adverse reactions, side effects and service user and family education**
- **Working with older and younger service users**
- **Multi-professional working**

www.openup.co.uk

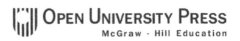

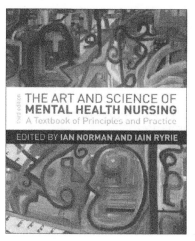

THE ART AND SCIENCE OF MENTAL HEALTH NURSING
A Textbook of Principles and Practice
Third Edition

Ian Norman and Iain Ryrie

ISBN: 9780335245611 (Paperback)
eBook: 9780335245628
2013

This well-established textbook is a must buy for all mental health nursing students. Comprehensive and broad, it explores in detail the many ways in which mental health nursing can have a positive impact on the lives of those with mental health problems. This book includes pedagogy to help students get the most out of each chapter and apply theory to practice in a rewarding way

Key features:

- **Case Studies:** Based on real practice in a variety of settings
- **Thinking Space:** These will help you reflect on your practice and assess your learning
- **Quotes from service users:** These offer the service user perspective throughout the book

www.openup.co.uk

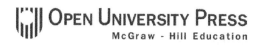

OPEN UNIVERSITY PRESS
McGraw - Hill Education

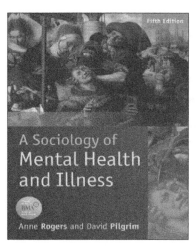

A SOCIOLOGY OF MENTAL HEALTH AND ILLNESS
Fifth Edition

Anne Rogers and David Pilgrim

ISBN: 9780335262762 (Paperback)
eBook: 9780335262779
2014

How do we understand mental health problems in their social context?
A former BMA Medical Book of the Year award winner, this book provides a
sociological analysis of major areas of mental health and illness. The book
considers contemporary and historical aspects of sociology, social
psychiatry, policy and therapeutic law to help students develop an in-depth
and critical approach to this complex subject.

Key features:

- Brand new chapter on prisons, criminal justice and mental health
- Expanded coverage of stigma, class and social networks
- Updated material on the Mental Capacity Act, Mental Health Act and
  the Deprivation of Liberty

www.openup.co.uk

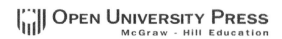